endometriosis
& OTHER PELVIC PAIN

A COMPREHENSIVE GUIDE
TO ALL TREATMENT OPTIONS

Dr Susan Evans

PIATKUS

Copyright © 2005 by Dr Susan F Evans

First published in 2005 by
Thomas C Lothian Pty Ltd

First published in Great Britain in 2006 by
Piatkus Books Ltd
5 Windmill Street, London W1T 2JA
email: info@piatkus.co.uk

The moral right of the author has been asserted

A catalogue record for this book is available from the British Library

ISBN 0 7499 2705 4

Text design by Patrick Cannon
Illustrations by Kathryn Skelsey

This book has been printed on paper manufactured
with respect for the environment using wood from
managed sustainable resources

Data manipulation by
Action Publishing Technology Ltd, Gloucester
Printed and bound in Great Britain by
MPG Books, Bodmin, Cornwall

Contents

Note
Words in the text that appear in bold, e.g. **laparoscopy**
are defined in the glossary.

Acknowledgments

M EDICINE DID NOT teach me how to write, so were it not for the guiding assistance of Julie Stanton, and Lois Grant, I am not sure this book would ever have been finished. It would certainly not have happened without the support of the women who keep my life together: Diana Morgan, Kathleen Connelly, and Deborah Adam.

I am very grateful for Margaret Taylor and Jane Marsh's contributions. Without them it would not be the well-rounded book we hope it to be. Thank you.

My medical colleagues Drs Anne Corbould, Jill Benson, Claire Fairweather, Helena Frawley, Jenny Cook, David Redwine, Penny Briscoe, Neil Hotham, Samantha Pillay, Larry Demco, Christine Kirby, Jane Andrews, Wayne Gillett, Fiona Stewart, Katrina Allen, Nesrin Varol, Susan Treloar, and Mark Arens all generously gave their time providing or reviewing the information.

Danielle Drever, John, Phoebe and Jack Allison, Rowena and Michael Vnuk, Joan Evans, Diana Morgan, Lata and Asha Mayer, David, Topsy and John Evans, Leith Banney, Patricia Johnson, Pat Griffiths, Lynne Mitchell, Peter and Betty Dawson, Barbara Dalwood, Belinda and Kelly Loveless, and Anne-Marie Ramsay read the book and offered kind words of very welcome criticism.

Serono Australia kindly provided the illustration on which Fig 5.1 is based, and Schering kindly allowed us to reproduce the Mirena device shown in Fig 6.3.

From a personal perspective, I would like to thank Maureen Merrick, Thembi Mazeka, Sharon Whitelaw-Jenkins, Draga Tomich, Rob Laing and Graham Van Renen; the best surgical team I could hope for, and Dr Ossie Petrucco who started me on the road to laparoscopic surgery. I would also like to thank Sheryl Klingner, Thom Rebner and Nick Warden who have supported our endometriosis clinic at Burnside War Memorial Hospital from the beginning.

However, most of all, I would like to thank my patients, who have trusted me with their endometriosis surgery over several years. Thank you.

Check with your doctor

The information in this book is intended only as a guide to help you when you are diagnosed with endometriosis, or suffer other types of pelvic pain. Neither the author nor the publisher can accept responsibility for your health or any decisions you make regarding your condition, or the treatments you choose. I would urge you to discuss your own special situation with your doctor and take their advice into account before you decide on any particular treatment.

Dedication

To my parents, Topsy and David, who have always encouraged me, and to my husband, John, with much love and many thanks.

Introduction

WOMEN FIND OUT they have endometriosis in many ways. Some realise early that there is something wrong and look for help. Others have endometriosis found unexpectedly during investigation for pelvic pain, an ovarian cyst that hasn't gone away or difficulty becoming pregnant.

As most people in the community know very little about endometriosis, few women recognise what their pain might mean. You may have had your pain for many years believing it to be normal, or due to another condition such as irritable bowel syndrome. Finding out that your pain is actually 'endometriosis' may be a relief that your pain has a name, or a cause for anger and disappointment that the diagnosis took so long.

It would be really nice if endometriosis was easy to diagnose, but it isn't. There is no one problem that all women with endometriosis share and we are not born with a label saying endometriosis! It can only be seen clearly at an operation called a **laparoscopy**, where a telescope is inserted through a small cut near the navel to view the inside of the pelvis. This is the operation most commonly used to diagnose and treat endometriosis.

As an endometriosis surgeon, I am very conscious that not *all* pelvic pain is due to endometriosis. Newer surgical techniques can greatly improve and sometimes cure pain in women where endometriosis is the *only* cause for their pain. However, even the best surgery will not be enough for women with a mixture of different pelvic pains. These women may leave their gynaecologist disappointed with what their endometriosis treatment has achieved for them. Endometriosis was only part of the problem and it is easy to feel that your carers have lost interest in your needs. Your problems have become just too hard for them to manage.

The best endometriosis care combines best quality surgery, a thorough search for other causes of pelvic pain, emotional support through the personal problems women with endometriosis may suffer and a recognition that complementary therapies can play a useful role. This is the care only a team can provide — individualised and sensitive to each woman's needs and preferences.

So what can this book do for you?

First, it sets out the facts about endometriosis and other types of pelvic pain as we know them to date. Second, it provides the knowledge you need to be actively involved with your doctor in choosing your own care. Throughout the book, I have included the stories of real women I have cared for with their names and some details changed for privacy.

Chapters 1, 2, and 3 provide basic information: What is endometriosis? Could I have endometriosis? How is endometriosis diagnosed? Even women with a long history of endometriosis will find something new and useful here.

Chapter 4 provides a history of endometriosis management over the last 30 years. Thankfully a lot has changed. Young women will find it interesting and appreciate how treatment has improved, but older women may recognise their own experience.

Chapter 5 describes what a laparoscopy is, how to prepare for one, what it can show and what the risks are. Many women have had a laparoscopy, but few understand what it involves.

Chapter 6 outlines the medicines used to treat endometriosis. It also describes how to use common pain medications effectively, and manage your periods.

Chapter 7 looks at the situations you may be in yourself. Whether you are a teenager with period pain, a woman who has 'tried everything', or a woman with endometriosis in the family, there are sections for you.

Chapter 8 answers the questions women often ask at our endometriosis clinic. Will I be able to have children? Will I need a hysterectomy? Will it turn to cancer?

Chapter 9 describes other causes of pelvic pain, what you can do about them and who can help you. You may recognise your own pain from among them. If so it will shorten your path to the right diagnosis and the treatment you need.

A good relationship with the people we choose to care for us is important. Chapter 10 explains how to choose a gynaecologist, what questions to ask and how to prepare for your visit.

In Chapter 11 Jane Marsh, the endometriosis nurse counsellor with whom I work, provides coping strategies and practical advice for women and their partners. Treating the whole woman means looking at all the aspects of her life that contribute to her total pain experience.

In Chapter 12 Dr Margaret Taylor, specialist in nutritional and herbal medicines, describes how these treatments relate to endo-metriosis. There is practical advice on how to balance your hormones and manage premenstrual syndrome.

Twenty years ago, women with pelvic pain were thought to have emotional problems rather than a medical condition. This reflected our lack of knowledge at that time. Looking back, many of these women had undiagnosed endometriosis. There is more to offer now. Fewer women have undiagnosed pain, and far fewer are told that their pain is normal.

We hope this book helps you.

SUSAN EVANS

Chapter 1

....

What is endometriosis?

EVEN WOMEN WHO have known of their endometriosis for many years may be unsure what endometriosis actually is. That is understandable. Doctors find it confusing too.

Endometriosis is a condition where bits of tissue that are similar to the lining of the uterus are found in places outside the uterus where they shouldn't be. This tissue is *not* the same as the lining of the uterus, but it looks similar under a microscope.

Areas of endometriosis are called **lesions**. Lesion is just a medical word for any area of abnormality. A mole on your skin, or a wart on your hand can also be called a lesion.

Endometriosis is a problem because it can cause pain and scarring.

What does endometriosis look like?

Most endometriosis is found in the **pelvis**. Endometriosis lesions form a spotty covering on the side walls of the pelvis, or on the surface of the pelvic organs. These organs include the uterus, ovaries, fallopian tubes, bladder, bowel, **ureter** and appendix. More severe endometriosis grows into the pelvic organs themselves.

Figure 1.1 The pelvic organs seen from the front

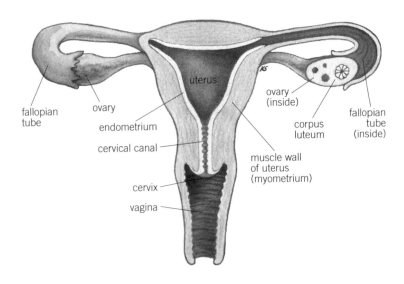

Figure 1.2 The pelvic organs seen through a laparoscope

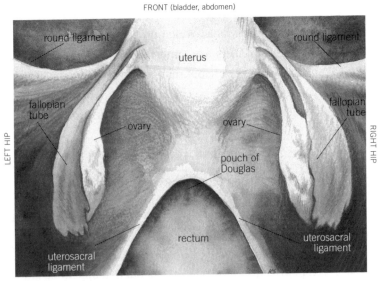

What your pelvis looks like through a laparoscope

At school you learned about what the pelvic organs look like from the front (see Fig 1.1). This is useful for many things, but not showing endometriosis. Endometriosis lies on the surface of organs not inside them, which is why the pictures in this book look different from those you may be used to. They show what your surgeon sees when he or she looks at your pelvis through the laparoscope. If you are shown pictures of your pelvis after your surgery, these are the type of pictures you will see, so you need to understand what they show (see Fig 1.2).

Imagine that you are looking down at your own pelvis through your navel. You will see the pelvic organs from above. In the middle lies the uterus. On either side there is an ovary, and a fallopian tube. Behind the uterus, the uterosacral ligaments extend from the back of the uterus to the back of the pelvis around the pouch of Douglas. The rectum (lower part of the bowel) passes through the centre of the pouch of Douglas and the ureters lie in the pelvic sidewall on both sides. In front of the uterus is the bladder.

All the organs you can see are covered by peritoneum (thin skin) and this is where any endometriosis will lie. Figure 1.2 shows a normal pelvis. Other pictures in the book show a laparoscopy (page 40), an endometrioma (page 45), and an adhesion (page 16).

As both the pelvic organs and the side walls of the pelvis are covered with a thin slippery skin called **peritoneum**, it is in the peritoneum that most endometriosis is found.

Endometriosis lesions come in many colours, shapes and sizes, some easier to recognise than others (see Reference 1). These different colours probably reflect different stages in the development of endometriosis. They include:

- *Red lesions.* These are red because they contain many blood vessels. They look like small red lumps or maybe just a group of blood vessels in one spot. Red lesions may be the first stage of endometriosis.
- *Clear lesions.* These look like tiny bubbles. They are another form of early endometriosis and can be quite difficult to see.
- *Black lesions.* Endometriosis irritates the peritoneum around it causing scarring. Any blood trapped in the scar tissue turns black.
- *White lesions.* Over time, the scarring around the endometriosis blocks any blood vessels. The body absorbs the black colour, leaving a thick white scar.
- *Endometriomas* or *chocolate cysts.* These are larger lumps of endometriosis that grow inside an ovary (see page 45).
- *Peritoneal windows or pockets.* These are oval-shaped areas that look like a dent in the surface. For many years no-one understood what peritoneal windows were. However, small samples (biopsies) of these 'windows' sent to a pathologist and checked through a microscope often show endometriosis.
- *Invisible areas.* Sometimes biopsies taken from peritoneum that looks normal show tiny (microscopic) areas of endometriosis. This is particularly common if the biopsy is taken close to obvious areas of endometriosis.

Young women are more likely to have clear, pink or red lesions. These are the most active forms of endometriosis and the lesions most likely to cause pain. Unfortunately they are also the most difficult lesions to recognise at a **laparoscopy**. Older women usually have white, brown or black lesions. They have probably been present for longer.

Most endometriosis lesions are thin and small – maybe 1 or 2 mm across. Larger and thicker lesions are called *nodules*. These are usually a few millimetres to a few centimetres across.

Chocolate cysts are the largest form of endometriosis. They may be several centimetres across. The word *cyst* just means a space with fluid inside it. It is the type of cells around the edge of a cyst (the lining) that tells what type of cyst it is. The lining of an **endometrioma** is made up of cells that look like the lining of the uterus. The fluid inside the cyst is dark brown and looks a lot like chocolate sauce. This is why they are called chocolate cysts.

If a woman has only a few endometriosis lesions, her condition is described as *mild* endometriosis. Her endometriosis may never be a problem for her. It may have been found by accident during an operation for another reason, such as a sterilisation procedure in women who have completed their families. If she has many lesions, or the lesions are large, her condition is called *severe* endometriosis. *Moderate* endometriosis is therefore somewhere between the two.

Although almost all endometriotic lesions are found in the pelvis, sometimes they are found in unusual places such as the **navel** (also called the umbilicus or belly button), an old caesarean section scar, or the lungs. Very rarely, they have been found in men who have used oesatrogen hormone medication.

Although endometriosis is especially common in Western countries, it can be found throughout the world and among women of all ethnic backgrounds.

The good news is that although it can spread, *endometriosis is not a cancer.*

Why is it called endometriosis?

The word endometriosis comes from the word **endometrium**. Endometrium is the medical name for the lining of the uterus (womb). 'Endo' means inside and 'metra' means uterus. It is the endometrium that grows inside the uterus each month, and then bleeds away during a period. Although they look similar through a microscope, an area of endometriosis is *not* the same as the lining of the uterus. Endometri*osis* lesions rarely bleed and make different hormones than normal endometri*um*.

How does endometriosis cause pain?

No-one knows exactly why endometriosis causes pain. It can certainly cause pain if it makes an ovary stick to other organs in the pelvis. This is called an **adhesion**. However, many women with endometriosis have pain but no adhesions.

What *is* known is that endometriosis lesions make many chemical substances that can cause irritation or scarring of the tissue around them. It may be these chemicals that cause the pain. Deeper areas of endometriosis may press on tiny nerves in the pelvis causing pain. This is especially likely if the endometriosis involves the **uterosacral ligaments** (see Chapter 2, page 14).

It is commonly said that endometriosis lesions cause pain because they bleed during a period and the trapped blood has nowhere to go. However, as many painful endometriosis lesions don't bleed, this is unlikely to be true in most cases.

Could J have endometriosis?

YES. ANY WOMAN OLD ENOUGH to have periods could have endometriosis, but luckily most don't. Around one in ten women will develop endometriosis at some time during their life, but as much of this is mild endometriosis they may never realise it is there, and it may never be a problem.

What symptoms fit with endometriosis?

Symptoms are health problems you notice when you are unwell. For example, a runny nose, headache and fever are symptoms of a cold, and painful joints are symptoms of arthritis. This chapter describes the common symptoms of endometriosis in detail. It explains how to tell if these symptoms might mean endometriosis.

The commonest symptoms of endometriosis are:

- Painful periods (see page 13)
- Pain at ovulation (see page 15)
- Pelvic pain between periods (see page 17)

- Painful sex (see page 19)
- Pain opening bowels (see page 21)
- Bleeding between periods (see page 22)
- Difficulty becoming pregnant (see page 23)
- Pain passing urine (see page 24)
- Tiredness (see page 24)
- Unusual symptoms (see page 25)

Luckily very few women have all these symptoms. While most have pain, others have no pain. Some find it difficult to become pregnant, whereas others conceive easily. If you do have endometriosis, your particular symptoms will depend on where in your pelvis the endometriosis is. The symptoms of endometriosis vary so much that few women have the same experience.

If you do have any of these symptoms, it does not mean that you definitely have endometriosis. There are so many other conditions that cause similar problems that it may be due to something else. The only reliable way to diagnose endometriosis is with a laparoscopy, but as no-one wants an operation they don't need it is a good idea to think about what else it might be before booking your surgery. There may be another explanation for your pain, and you may want to try medications, or have other tests first.

For example, most teenagers have period pain but less than one in ten has endometriosis. It is not reasonable to do a laparoscopy on all teenage girls with period pain, yet some need one. Trying other treatments first, and leaving a laparoscopy for those teenagers for whom other treatments don't help saves a lot of surgery on otherwise healthy young women (see Chapter 7, page 87).

Your general practitioner can help you work through this, but ultimately you are the one with the pain and you are the one best able to decide if you need a laparoscopy. So regardless of what your family, friends or doctor say, if your symptoms are a major problem to you, and other treatments have not helped, then look further. You may have endometriosis. Trust your own judgement.

Painful periods

Endometriosis anywhere in the pelvis can cause period pain (**dysmenorrhoea**) — it's the most common symptom. In fact, if you have period pain bad enough to seek a doctor's advice then you have around a 50 per cent chance of having endometriosis. The chance is even higher if you also have endometriosis in your family.

The other causes of period pain apart from endometriosis include pain from the uterus itself (Chapter 9, page 155) due to chemicals in the uterus called prostaglandins, **adenomyosis** (Chapter 9, page 151) due to changes like endometriosis in the wall of the uterus, and clot colic (Chapter 9, page 158) in women with very heavy, clotty periods. You may have more than one cause for your period pain.

Prostaglandins cause the 'normal' period pain that young women suffer before having their first baby. Although called 'normal', this downplays just how severe the pain may be. Prostaglandin pain usually comes at the beginning of a period. It should only last for one or two days and is much better on the contraceptive pill or with normal period pain medications such as Ibuprofen or Naproxen (Chapter 6, page 63). If your pain goes away with any of these medications then you have prostaglandin period pain and your chance of having endometriosis is low. Period pain medications need to be taken correctly if they are to work well. There are instructions on how to take them in Chapter 6 on page 63.

Endometriosis period pain usually lasts longer than a day. There may be pain leading up to, or right through a period. Period pain in the lower back is especially common in women with endometriosis near the uterosacral ligaments. These ligaments pass from the uterus back to a part of the spine called the sacrum, which lies at the back of the pelvis (see Fig 1.2). While they may help relieve the pain a little, neither the contraceptive pill nor period pain medications usually get rid of endometriosis pain.

Adenomyosis period pain is more common in middle-aged rather than young women, although this is not always true. It causes pain similar to endometriosis, but no endometriosis is found when a laparoscopy is done. The uterus is often a little enlarged. Gynaecologists use the word 'bulky' for a slightly enlarged uterus.

Will my pain get better if I have a baby?

Young women with period pain are often told not to worry because 'You will be fine once you have had a baby'. This may be true of prostaglandin pain, but is *not* true for the pain of endometriosis or adenomyosis. It is also small comfort for women who don't plan to have children. Pregnancy is a poor treatment for endometriosis. If you have already had a baby and your period pain is still severe it is quite likely that you have either endometriosis or adenomyosis.

So one way to tell whether you may have endometriosis is to treat pain from the uterus with medication such as the oral contraceptive pill or period pain medications and see whether you still have pain. If your pain goes away on either medication then endometriosis is still possible, but less likely. If it does not go away, endometriosis is more likely and the decision to have a laparoscopy may be easier for you. It is time to discuss your pain with a gynaecologist.

If you prefer to avoid using the contraceptive pill long term, just two months of treatment is enough to see if it helps your pain. After two months you can stop the Pill if you prefer. Your pain will return, but you may feel reassured that the chance of endometriosis is low.

Remember that endometriosis can occur at any age after periods begin. Teenagers are definitely *not* too young to have endometriosis.

J thought all women had pain like mine

Pauline is a 35-year-old married accountant who has chosen not to have children. She suffered severe period pain each month for many years despite the contraceptive pill and period pain medication. Pauline was very determined to cope and never missed a day at work, even if that meant using strong pain relief just to get through the day. Pauline thought that all women had pain like hers, so she never sought help. Finally the pain became so severe that she made an appointment to discuss an operation to remove her uterus (hysterectomy). We decided to look for endometriosis first. The laparoscopy showed extensive endometriosis, which was completely removed. Pauline was very pleased. The mild pain she still had with periods could now be managed with normal period pain medication, and she still had her uterus. Her concern was for the many women who, like her, do not seek treatment because they believe that their pain is normal.

Ovulation pain

Ovulation is the time of the month when an egg is released from an ovary. Some pain at ovulation may be normal, but if so it should only last for a day, swap sides approximately every second month, and be much better with period pain medications. This type of pain is called *mittelschmerz* (it means 'middle pain' in German).

Contraceptive pills that stop ovulation should stop **ovulation pain**, so be suspicious if you notice ovulation pain while you're on the Pill. There is information on how to work out when you ovulate in Chapter 8 on page 123.

Sometimes endometriosis forms scar tissue that sticks the pelvic organs together. The places where the organs are stuck together are called *adhesions*. Adhesions or endometriosis near an ovary can tie the ovary to the side wall of the pelvis, causing ovulation pain that is *not* normal (see Figure 2.1, below).

If you have pain on one side of your pelvis with periods *and* at ovulation time, you may have endometriosis near that ovary. Ovulation pain on both sides of the pelvis at once may mean adhesions or endometriosis near both ovaries. To make it even more complicated, there are some women who have *crossover*

Figure 2.1 Adhesions

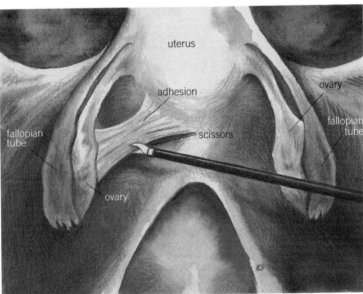

An adhesion between the left ovary and the uterus. Tiny scissors can be used to divide the adhesion and free the ovary.

pain. This is pain felt on one side of the pelvis, when the actual problem is on the other side.

> ### Period pain and ovulation pain
>
> Aisha is a 23-year-old university student with no children, nor any need for contraception. She had severe period pain for every day of her period even with period pain medications. Each month at ovulation she also suffered two or three days of pain on her left side. A laparoscopy showed endometriosis and adhesions tying down the left ovary. The right ovary was normal. The left ovary was freed and the endometriosis removed. After her operation, Aisha's period pain was much better. She still had pain on the first day of her period, but this was now easily treated with period pain medications. The ovulation pain on her left was gone.
>
> Before her surgery, Aisha had both endometriosis and prostaglandin pain. After her surgery only the prostaglandin pain remained.

Pelvic pain between periods

While women who only have pain with periods can do their best to 'live with' the pain and plan their life around those days, it is very hard to live with pain present on most days that can come at any time. What is more, the longer you do 'live with it' the more it affects your work, education, relationships, mood, self-esteem and general health. If you have this type of pain, it may or may not be endometriosis, but you do need to work on a solution.

How can I tell if these pains are endometriosis?

Pain between periods that is due to endometriosis usually feels similar to period pain. It may not be as bad as your period pain, but it feels similar in quality. As a period comes closer, the pain usually becomes more severe and more frequent. The week after your period should be your best time of the month. Pain felt in one particular spot, that follows this pattern, is often endometriosis.

If your pain comes at any time of the month, regardless of when your period is due, then it is probably something else. Remember that you may have a mixture of endometriosis *and* another condition. As pain starting in the bladder, bowel, muscles, ligaments, uterus or pelvic nerves all travels to the brain through similar pathways, it is hard for your brain to separate out all the different pains and decide where each pain came from. Many different pains can feel similar.

Treating endometriosis can only help those symptoms that are due to endometriosis. It is an important first step, but pains from other organs will remain unless they are treated too.

But J have pain all the time!

Pain almost every day over a long period of time is called *chronic pain*. Chronic pain is enough to wear anyone down. It is miserable. It is also something that we as doctors do not know enough about. If you have chronic pain, your situation is complicated but certainly not hopeless. Knowledge about what causes chronic pelvic pain has improved greatly. As time goes by, more and more of what could not be diagnosed in the past has a name. Women knew all along that there was something wrong with them. Sure they were stressed. They had chronic pain!

To me, there is rarely one simple cause (or solution) for this type of pain. Endometriosis is usually only part of the picture. This is why the sections on pages 107 and 143 have been written. If you can recognise yourself in any of the descriptions in Chapter 9, it will be easier to decide where to go for help. A laparoscopy will only be part of the treatment you need. Other types of pain need their own care.

Painful sex

Painful intercourse (**dyspareunia**) is common in women with endometriosis. As well as the physical pain, there is the emotional pain and guilt that women feel when they are unable to enjoy sex with their partner. No one feels like sex if they know it will hurt.

There are many other causes of painful sex apart from endometriosis, so the best person to see first is your general practitioner. Endometriosis rarely causes pain near the opening of the vagina and does *not* cause vaginal itching, a smelly vaginal discharge or vulval skin irritation. These problems are due to other conditions. Skin conditions of the vulva (checked by biopsy and examination), troublesome vaginal muscle contractions (*vaginismus*), vaginal infections ('thrush'), an irritated bladder (see Chapter 9, page 188), or occasionally a uterus that lies at the back of the pelvis (retroverted uterus) can all make sex painful. Your general practitioner can check for some of these causes. A difficult relationship with your partner may also be a factor.

Vaginismus can be treated, but is not something that an operation will fix. It happens when sex has been painful for some time. The muscles at the opening of the vagina tighten any time that sex is attempted. You will not be able to 'just relax' (even if you want to) and stop it happening. In most larger cities, there is a doctor who specialises in sex counselling for couples. They can help your vaginismus. If intercourse has been painful for some time, you and your partner may have many issues to work through to regain a satisfying sexual relationship.

Painful intercourse due to endometriosis is felt deep inside the pelvis. It may be worse in some sexual positions (depending on where the endometriosis is) and can last for one or two days afterwards. Dyspareunia is especially common when the endometriosis lies behind the uterus near the top of the vagina. This area includes the *pouch of Douglas*, the uterosacral ligaments, and the *recto-vaginal septum*, which can be seen in Figure 5.1 on page 40.

An operation to remove endometriosis from here may be difficult because it is close to the bowel. Other options include a Mirena IUD (see Chapter 6, page 77), or a progestogen medication (see Chapter 6, page 75). If sex is still painful after *all* your endometriosis has been removed, there may be another reason for your pain.

Who was Douglas, and why was the pouch named after him?

James Douglas lived in England from 1675 to 1742. He is described as a 'man-midwife' (gynaecologist) and physician to the queen. His particular interest was the structure of the human body (anatomy). He described the area of the pelvis between the back of the uterus and the lower bowel that we now call the pouch of Douglas. When seen through a laparoscope it is the deepest part of the pelvis. It is also a common place to find endometriosis.

Endometriosis with painful sex — Case 1

Joanne is a married woman of 30 with two young children. Neither her periods nor sex had been a problem for her in the past, but over two years she had noticed pain with intercourse. She described the pain as being in one spot, deep inside and a little to the left. She was exactly right! At her laparoscopy, there was a nodule of endometriosis in the left uterosacral ligament between the uterus and the bowel. The rest of her pelvis was normal. The nodule was removed and her pain was gone.

Endometriosis with painful sex — Case 2

Jacinta is a 25-year-old married university student. Despite periods that were only mildly uncomfortable, and a strong relationship with her husband, intercourse had always been painful. A laparoscopy showed endometriosis in the pouch of Douglas, behind the uterus. The endometriosis was removed but her pain only partially improved. Much of her pain was found to be a vaginal skin condition.

Pain opening or bleeding from the bowels

The bowel lies very close to the uterus, fallopian tubes and ovaries. It is also a common place to find endometriosis. Because of this, it is not surprising that many women with endometriosis have bowel problems, especially at period time. Sorting out how much of the problem is due to the bowel itself and how much is due to endometriosis can be very difficult. There is more information on irritable bowel syndrome in Chapter 9 on page 161.

Endometriosis near the bowel may be difficult to remove surgically. It may also be difficult to see during a laparoscopy because it hides below the surface of the peritoneum. Sometimes it is easier to see (or feel) as a lump (nodule) in the back wall of the vagina. Most women with endometriosis here will have bowel pain, back pain and painful intercourse.

When bleeding from the bowel occurs at period time it is more likely to be due to extra blood vessels in the bowel wall than endometriosis that has grown through the wall of the bowel. It may also be due to other conditions such as haemorrhoids, bowel disease or occasionally a cancer. So if you have bleeding from the bowel you should tell your general practitioner straightaway.

It is important *not* to assume that the bleeding is due to endometriosis until you are sure that other conditions have been excluded.

My laparoscopy only showed 'mild' endometriosis but lots of scar tissue near the bowel. So why do I have so much pain?

Endometriosis lesions are often found in particular patterns. One of these patterns involves endometriosis in both uterosacral ligaments and the pouch of Douglas (see Figure 1.2 on page 6). There may be only a few brown lesions found (which is why it is mistaken for 'mild' endometriosis), but lots of white scarring on the uterosacral ligaments. The ovaries are often normal. These women usually have back pain, pain with intercourse and pain when opening their bowels. *This endometriosis is not 'mild' at all.* The white scarring is often endometriosis too. Removing this type of endometriosis requires a skilled endometriosis surgeon. It is difficult and can be dangerous. The good news is that completely removing *all* the scar tissue, often with some of the uterosacral ligaments, usually makes a big difference to the pain.

Bleeding between periods (intermenstrual bleeding)

No one knows why bleeding between periods is common in women with endometriosis, but as the endometriosis lesions produce so many hormones and chemicals, it is not surprising that bleeding happens sometimes. If the amount of blood is small, it is called *spotting*.

Before presuming that your bleeding is due to endometriosis, other causes of bleeding need to be excluded. Your general practitioner can help you with this. The contraceptive pill, an unexpected pregnancy or soft fleshy lumps called *polyps* can all cause bleeding between periods. Very occasionally, bleeding between periods is a sign of cancer of the cervix or uterus so you must make sure that your cervical smear tests are up to date and you may also need an ultrasound scan to check the lining of the uterus.

> **Bleeding between periods is not normal, so you should always discuss it with your doctor.**

If the bleeding *is* due to endometriosis, it is more likely in the week before a period than the week after a period. You may have tried several types of contraceptive pill, hoping to find one that didn't cause bleeding between periods, only to find later that endometriosis was the cause of the bleeding, not the Pill. Once the endometriosis is removed, the spotting usually improves.

Difficulty falling pregnant (infertility)

Most of us expect that when we decide to become pregnant, it will happen. Few conditions are more distressing than infertility. As well as the pain of endometriosis, there is the disappointment as each period arrives. There may also be a feeling of guilt at 'letting down' your partner.

While endometriosis *is* more common among women who have difficulty becoming pregnant, this does not mean that all women with endometriosis are infertile. Many women with endo-metriosis become pregnant easily. What it does mean is that endometriosis is one factor that *may* affect your fertility. It is one factor not in your favour. However, it takes two to become pregnant and there are many factors that affect fertility (both yours and your partner's). If all the other factors are normal, you may never have a problem.

Those women with endometriosis who do have problems becoming pregnant often have either more severe endometriosis or there are other factors involved. There is more information about endometriosis and fertility in Chapter 8 on page 119.

> If you don't want to become pregnant, then reliable
> contraception is just as important for you as any
> other woman.

Pain or bleeding passing urine (dysuria)

Most **dysuria** is due to problems with the bladder itself rather than
endometriosis. These bladder problems include bladder infections
and another condition called *interstitial cystitis* (IC) (see Chapter 9
on page 188). Both can cause pain in the lower **abdomen** or make
you want to pass urine more often (**frequency**).

It is true that endometriosis can cause these problems too, but
unless you have other reasons to believe you have endometriosis
(like painful periods), it is best to talk to your general practitioner
or a bladder doctor (urologist) about your bladder. A laparoscopy
looking for endometriosis is only necessary if they are unable to
help you and endometriosis seems possible.

No one knows why, but many women with endometriosis
also have interstitial cystitis. This is one reason why some women
may be disappointed with their endometriosis treatment. Some
of their symptoms improved once the endometriosis was
removed, but their bladder symptoms remained. A laparoscopy
will not help IC: it needs its own treatment plan (see Chapter 9,
page 188).

Occasionally endometriosis grows on the inside of the bladder
itself. About one in five of these women will notice blood in their
urine at period time.

Tiredness

There is no easy explanation why women with endometriosis often
feel tired. It may be that whenever the body is unwell in some way,
energy is the first thing to fail. Pain itself is very wearing. So are the

worry and stress involved in trying to maintain a normal life and normal relationships despite pain. Chapter 11, written by Jane Marsh, looks at ways to live better with your pain.

Unusual symptoms

The symptoms that I have described so far cover almost all endometriosis. Occasionally endometriosis is found in unusual places and can cause unusual symptoms. For example:

- Pain just below the ribs, worse on breathing in, and only present with periods might be endometriosis of the **diaphragm**. It is rare.
- Pain in one part of a caesarean section scar that is much worse with periods may be due to endometriosis in the scar. It is uncommon.
- Pain down the back of the leg (sciatica) present only during periods, might be endometriosis of the sciatic nerve. It is very rare indeed.
- A lump in the navel that is tender at period time may be endometriosis of the navel. It is uncommon.

Endometriosis in unusual places is painful at the time of a period because no matter where it is, it still responds to the normal hormonal changes of the menstrual cycle. However, these examples are rare.

> Women with endometriosis have symptoms that other people can't see and don't understand. Even friends and relatives who are kind, caring and patient may become frustrated when your symptoms don't improve. No matter how kind, considerate and caring you partner is, he has never had period pain. Other women with trouble-free periods may wonder why your periods should be

such a problem, and be very unsympathetic. It is therefore not surprising that many women with undiagnosed endometriosis lose faith in their ability to judge their pain. They wonder whether the pain is normal or they are just weak.

Trust your own judgement and ask your doctor about endometriosis if you believe this could be the cause of your pain. You may need to ask more than one doctor to find the help you need.

Chapter 3

How is endometriosis diagnosed?

L IFE WOULD BE MUCH SIMPLER if endometriosis was easy to diagnose. There are no blood tests that diagnose it reliably and most women with endometriosis will have a normal ultrasound scan. The only reliable way to diagnose or exclude endometriosis is a laparoscopy done by a gynaecologist who is experienced in recognising endometriosis. This is a big step for many women, and one that should not be taken without reason. Then again, most women with severe pelvic pain *do* have good reason. Their pain is severe. I find that a woman who requests a laparoscopy because she is concerned about her pelvic pain is usually right.

What can a laparoscopy show?

A laparoscopy can show whether endometriosis is present, where it is and how severe it is. It also allows removal of the endometriosis at the same time or at least a plan for removal of the endometriosis on another day.

A laparoscopy where no endometriosis is found is not wasted

effort. Many women are less concerned about their pain once they know that their pelvic organs are healthy. A normal laparoscopy may have excluded endometriosis as a cause for the pain, but does *not* mean that the pain does not exist. It does, but it's now time to move on and consider other possible causes (see Chapter 9).

You should never be disappointed with a normal laparoscopy. A normal pelvis is *always* the best outcome.

What can an ultrasound show?

Most endometriosis does *not* show on an ultrasound scan. The endometriosis lesions are too thin. An ultrasound scan will show the size of an ovary clearly, but not whether it has spots on its surface. As most endometriosis changes the surface appearance of pelvic organs, rather than their size, most ultrasound scans in women with endometriosis are normal.

One form of endometriosis that *is* large enough to show on an ultrasound scan is an endometrioma, or chocolate cyst (see Figure 5.2, page 45). The 'chocolate sauce' inside the cyst gives it a special appearance on an ultrasound scan. The cyst looks like ground glass, which means that it has a grainy look. This appearance on an ultrasound usually means one of two things:

- That you have an endometrioma, or
- That you have a type of cyst called a *haemorrhagic corpus luteum.*

A corpus luteum is the normal cyst that an ovary makes each month after ovulation, and the word 'haemorrhagic' means that it has blood inside. This type of cyst goes away by itself. So, if you have a cyst on ultrasound scan with a grainy, ground-glass appearance, then time will tell what type of cyst it is likely to be. A haemorrhagic corpus luteum will usually go away by itself within three months, whereas an endometrioma will not. If your cyst is still there at a second scan done two or three months later, then your cyst is probably an endometrioma, and you should discuss it with a gynaecologist. The endometrioma may need to be removed, but depending on your particular situation and wishes, the ovary can usually be saved.

An American study (see Reference 2) showed that if an endometrioma can be seen on an ultrasound scan, it is 99 per cent likely that there will be other areas of endometriosis present too. These other areas may not show on a scan, but they *are* there. So, if you have a laparoscopy to remove an endometrioma from your ovary, you should expect that other areas of endometriosis could be found too.

An ultrasound scan is also useful in women with pelvic problems because it may show other conditions such as **fibroids** in the uterus or ovarian cysts that are unrelated to endometriosis.

What can blood tests show?

There is *no* blood test that will reliably diagnose endometriosis. Occasionally blood is taken to check the amount of a substance called CA-125 in the blood. Many different pelvic conditions, including endometriosis can make the CA-125 level a little high. However, as a normal CA-125 result does not exclude endometriosis, this test is only useful in special situations.

One of these special situations is where an ultrasound has shown an unusual looking ovarian cyst, especially in a woman over 40 years of age. Such a cyst may occasionally be a cancer of the ovary. A cancer of the ovary sometimes makes the CA-125 level very high. Unfortunately, it is not a reliable test for cancer either, because some women with cancer of the ovary have a normal CA-125 level.

A CA-125 is rarely useful in younger women, or women with normal looking ovaries on ultrasound scan.

Why did it take so long for my endometriosis to be diagnosed?

As all the symptoms of endometriosis may be due to other conditions, it is disappointing, but not surprising, that it may take years for a woman's endometriosis to be diagnosed. How many years? In Norway and Australia it takes an average of six years, and in the USA an average of nine years from the beginning of symptoms to diagnosis. This is a long time to have pain. In the USA studies, half the time was lost because women did not report their problems to their doctor, but the other half was medical time lost before a reliable laparoscopy was done (see References 3 and 4).

How is endometriosis of the bowel diagnosed?

The bowel is a long coiled-up tube running from your stomach to your anus. It has an inside and an outside. The outside of the lower bowel and the appendix can be seen at a laparoscopy. The inside of the lower bowel can only be seen by passing a flexible camera through the anus and up into the bowel. This procedure is called a *colonoscopy* and is usually only recommended in women with severe endometriosis that may have spread through the bowel wall, or in those women with other bowel symptoms.

As a laparoscopic surgeon, I am frequently surprised by what I find at a laparoscopy. Women with very few symptoms may have many endometriosis lesions, while others with many symptoms have a normal pelvis. So, how many symptoms you have or how severe your pain is may not be a reliable indicator of how much endometriosis you have.

| *Without a laparoscopy, you will never know.*

Chapter 4

. . . .

How has the management of endometriosis changed?

M ANY WOMEN ASK ME about the treatments they have had in
the past. Why weren't they offered better options earlier?
Why did it take so long to get a diagnosis? Generally I find that they
were offered the best that was available at the time. Treating
endometriosis effectively remains a challenge, but thankfully
improved treatments are now available.

A history of endometriosis treatment

Endometriosis in its most severe form has been known for centuries. From time to time, women had operations through large
cuts on their abdomen (a **laparotomy**), and chocolate cysts full of
dark brown fluid were found. Endometriosis was believed to be an
uncommon condition affecting women in their thirties and forties.

Before the 1970s, diagnosing pelvic pain was very difficult, particularly when no abnormality was found on examination. Neither
ultrasound scanning nor laparoscopy were available. If enlarged
ovaries were found on vaginal examination, then a large cut was

made in the abdomen to investigate the cause of the problem. If a chocolate cyst was found it was removed, together with part or all of an ovary. There was little else that could be done, particularly in women who hoped for a future pregnancy. Endometriosis in other areas of the pelvis was rarely removed because of the difficulty and dangers in doing so, and because many abnormalities we now know to be endometriosis were thought to be normal at that time.

It takes at least six weeks to recover from a laparotomy and fertility may be affected if adhesions form after the surgery. Because of this, gynaecologists were loath to operate on young women with pain, unless a specific lump was found on examination. They wished to avoid doing more harm than good.

As many women with endometriosis did not have a lump that could be felt at vaginal examination, most remained untreated. Understandably, women felt let down and angry when their pain was diagnosed and dismissed as emotional or bowel issues. Once childbearing was complete, many had an operation to remove the uterus (**hysterectomy**), frequently with both ovaries removed at the same time (**bilateral oophorectomy**). There was little else to offer.

Once laparoscopy became available in the 1970s and 1980s, pelvic pain could be investigated without a large cut, without risking fertility, and without a long hospital stay. The skills and instruments needed to remove even small areas of endometriosis through these small holes had not yet been developed, so a laparoscopy at that time gave only a look at the pelvis. If an abnormality were found, a large cut would be made to fix the problem. Even with this new tool to view the inside of the pelvis more easily, it took many years for gynaecologists to recognise what was normal and what was *not* normal. Laparoscopy gave a better, but different, view of the pelvis so there was a lot to learn.

Gynaecologists knew that chocolate cysts in the ovaries, and black lumps around the pelvis were endometriosis, but many other lesions were considered normal. If black or brown areas were seen at laparoscopy, many women were prescribed a six-month course of a medication called **danazol**, in an attempt to remove the endometriosis. Some women did well on danazol, especially those with mild endometriosis, but half of those treated suffered side effects that were too troublesome to continue the treatment.

After danazol came a group of medications that aimed at removing the endometriosis by turning off oestrogen production and creating a reversible menopause-like environment. These medications are called Gonadotrophin Releasing Hormone analogues or **GnRH analogues**. They include such medications as goserelin (Zoladex), leuprolide (Prostap) or nafarelin (Synarel).

I have patients who say they have never felt so good as when they were on GnRH analogues, and a few who have never felt better than when taking danazol, but side effects are often a problem. In addition, none of these medications treat large, scarred or deep areas of endometriosis effectively, and no endometriosis medications improve fertility.

During the 1980s and 1990s, gynaecologists started taking small samples of tissue called *biopsies* whenever they saw something unusual through the laparoscope. These biopsies were sent to a pathologist for diagnosis using a microscope. By the mid-1990s it became clear that many of these abnormalities were actually endometriosis. Endometriosis became a condition with variable appearance. The lesions could be clear, pink, red or white, as well as black or brown. Once these more subtle lesions were included, it became obvious that endometriosis was a lot more common than once thought. It was also recognised that endometriosis was a condition affecting young women as well as older women.

In the 1990s, as laparoscopic skills and instruments improved, techniques were developed to remove endometriosis, and so avoid the need for medication.

The first technique, and one still commonly used today, was electrocautery. **Cautery** uses an instrument to touch the top of the endometriosis lesion, and burn it with electricity. The lesion is 'cauterised' in the same way as a blood vessel that causes nose-bleeds may be cauterised. Cautery (sometimes called ablation) works best for small thin areas of endometriosis, particularly those on the ovary or uterus. Unfortunately, it often leaves deeper endometriosis untreated and may cause scar tissue. As endometriosis is often found near delicate organs, and the heat from cautery can spread further than desired, gynaecologists tend to *under*-cauterise rather than *over*-cauterise endometriosis lesions. This decreases the risk of damaging important pelvic structures, but does tend to leave some endometriosis behind. Women often feel better for a short time, but once the remaining endometriosis becomes active again, the pain may return.

Since the late 1990s, the emphasis has changed to **excisional surgery**. This means cutting out the endometriosis wherever possible. Excisional surgery aims to remove the endometriosis completely to decrease the chance of endometriosis recurrence and achieve a longer pain-free time. It takes longer to do and is technically more challenging than cautery, but it does mean that the endometriosis is removed completely. The surgeon can also operate closer to delicate organs such as the ureter (the long tube that carries urine from the kidney to the bladder), or the bowel. Even so, surgery in some areas, particularly those near the bowel or where extensive adhesions have glued the pelvic organs together, remains challenging even for experienced surgeons.

Excision surgery can be done with either electricity or *laser*. Laser has been used since the 1990s. It is not different surgery, rather a different way of doing the same thing. When used to *excise* rather than *cauterise (ablate)*, it is an effective treatment.

Theoretically, if all the endometriosis is removed, there should be less recurrence, better management of pain or fertility, and less need for medication.

All the above treatments are used today, although excisional surgery is currently considered the most effective treatment for endometriosis. Cautery, danazol, GnRH analogues and other medications still have a place in some situations. Excisional surgery has its problems too. It is major surgery through small holes. It has risks, and may cause scarring. In ten years' time, the treatments we are able to offer may be different again.

Current endometriosis management

None of us — whether we are surgeons, doctors who prefer to use medications, or complementary therapists — have all the answers. I like to think that we are closer to effective treatment now, but perfect treatments are still some way off.

As a surgeon who specialises in endometriosis, the treatments I recommend tend to be more surgically orientated. That does not mean that other treatments are not useful. They are. I offer medications to women whose endometriosis has not been completely removed, or those who have widespread but tiny thin lesions. We treat the other causes of pain so common in endometriosis (but so often missed), and our patients see a nurse counsellor for emotional support and lifestyle advice. Endometriosis is a complex condition and there is no 'right' way to treat everyone.

Regardless of treatment preference, most women with endometriosis will have an operation at some stage. This is because it is the only reliable way to diagnose endometriosis. My own philosophy is that if a laparoscopy is needed to diagnose the condition, why not remove the endometriosis at the same time? If this is possible then the medicines used to treat endometriosis described in Chapter 6 can usually be avoided.

However, depending on where you are, and the services available to you, the diagnosis and removal of endometriosis at the same time may not be possible. Sometimes, even if it is possible, it is not a good idea because the best conditions for your surgery may not be present. Surgery to remove endometriosis requires special surgical skills, specialised theatre staff, more operating theatre time, and specialised equipment. It is expensive care for a hospital to provide, even if a suitable surgeon is available. So, if time, personnel or equipment are not available, treatment is better planned as a two-step procedure. The first laparoscopy is done to see whether or not endometriosis is present, and to assess how severe the endometriosis is. The second laparoscopy is booked for a time when appropriate staff, equipment and theatre time are available for the endometriosis to be completely removed. This can work well, even if it is less convenient.

An alternative is one laparoscopy to diagnose the endometriosis, and then a trial of medication (see Chapter 6, page 68).

No matter how good the surgery, it cannot solve the other problems that women with endometriosis may have. Years of pain take their toll on a woman's emotional, employment, educational, relationship and sexual wellbeing. An operation, even if very successful, will not reverse this damage. However, effective surgery may be an opportunity to put some problems away and work on others.

The search for better, more effective and less intrusive treatment continues. So does the search for the cause of endometriosis, and ways to prevent it. Even so, endometriosis remains a challenge for both the women with the condition and the doctors who care for them.

What if I do nothing? Can endometriosis go away by itself?

Yes, especially if it is mild. An Australian study (see Reference 5) followed a group of women with endometriosis who each had two laparoscopies, done six months apart. Half the women had their endometriosis removed at the first laparoscopy. The other half had their endometriosis diagnosed but not removed until their second laparoscopy. None of the women knew which surgery they had had.

Of those women who had their endometriosis diagnosed but *not* removed at the first laparoscopy:

- 45 per cent had more endometriosis six months later
- 33 per cent had the same amount of endometriosis six months later, and
- 22 per cent had less endometriosis six months later.
  After the first laparoscopy, pain improved in:
- 80 per cent of the women who had had their endometriosis removed, but only
- 30 per cent of the women whose endometriosis had been diagnosed but not removed.

Twenty per cent had pain that did not improve even after their endometriosis was removed. These women certainly had endometriosis but there may have been another cause for their pain.

Can surgery fix all my pelvic pain?

Surgery to remove endometriosis will only help pain that is due to endometriosis. Surgery will not help pain due to other causes. So, if endometriosis is your *only* problem, then complete removal of the endometriosis may be able to help all your pain. However, I find that most women with endometriosis have more than one cause for their pain. So even the best surgery does not fix all their pain. It is more realistic to expect your pain to improve, or be easier to manage with medications after surgery, than for it to go completely.

The symptoms that are most likely to be due to endometriosis, and therefore most likely to improve after *complete* removal of endometriosis are:

- Pain during the month that feels like period pain
- Pain on opening your bowels, especially if this happens near your period
- Spotting between periods, if it is due to endometriosis
- Painful intercourse, if it is due to endometriosis

Pain during a period usually improves, but as this pain is usually a mixture of pains, it rarely goes away completely. Other possible causes of your pain are described in Chapter 9, and other treatments for period pain are included in Chapter 6 on pages 62 and 65.

Chapter 5

Laparoscopy

THIS CHAPTER EXPLAINS what a laparoscopy is and answers frequently asked questions about the procedure, how to prepare for the operation, and the risks and benefits involved.

What is a laparoscopy?

A laparoscopy may be the first operation you have ever had. Hospitals can be scary places to women who are unfamiliar with them. They don't need to be. The hospital staff are there to look after you, and both your anaesthetist and your gynaecologist will stay with you throughout your operation. Most operations go very smoothly.

A laparoscopy is done under a general anaesthetic, which means you will be asleep the whole time. Once you are asleep, a small cut is made near your navel and a telescope (called a *laparoscope*) is used to look inside and check your pelvis for any endometriosis.

Because the organs in the pelvis lie close together, a gas is used to inflate your abdomen and separate them. Without the gas, the pelvic organs could not be seen clearly. The cut near the navel

Figure 5.1 A laparoscopy

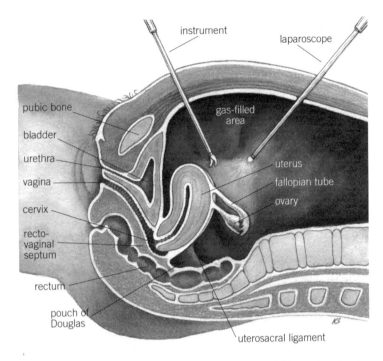

The laparoscope is inserted through a small cut near the navel. It is used to view the pelvic organs. The instruments used to remove endometriosis are inserted through small cuts lower down in the pelvis.

is used to view the pelvis, but if endometriosis is found inside, then more small cuts are needed. Between one and three extra cuts are made, so that the instruments needed to do your surgery can be inserted. What happens next depends on what has been found, and how your gynaecologist treats each problem.

Remember, it is not the small cuts on your abdomen that are the operation; it is what is done inside. Some laparoscopies are minor surgery, whereas other laparoscopies are major surgery through little holes.

After your laparoscopy, you will wake up in the *recovery ward*. This is a special area near the operating theatre where patients are cared for by nursing staff until they are more awake, and feeling comfortable. This usually takes one or two hours depending on what type of surgery you have had and how quickly you wake up. You will be attached to a saline drip (called an intravenous or IV drip) that provides water, salt and any medicine you need into one of the veins in your arm until you are able to eat and drink normally.

Any pieces of endometriosis that are removed during your operation will be sent to a pathologist, and checked with a microscope. This is because some lesions that look like endometriosis turn out to be something else, such as endosalpingiosis (see Chapter 9, page 203), inflammatory tissue, (see page 207) or scar tissue.

How long will my surgery take?

This also depends on what is found. If all looks normal, then your laparoscopy will usually take less than thirty minutes, whereas if you have severe endometriosis, it may take a few hours. Endometriosis surgery is delicate work using small instruments near sensitive structures, so it takes time.

How long will I need off work?

How long you stay in hospital, and have off school, work or normal activities depends on what type of work you do, what surgery was done, and how well you feel. A laparoscopy where nothing abnormal is found can usually be done as day surgery. This means that you are able to go home on the same day as your operation. However, you will still need between three and seven days off to recover.

If endometriosis *is* found at your laparoscopy and removed, the operation will take longer, and there will be more healing required. You will probably stay in hospital overnight, and may need one or two weeks off work.

If this is your first laparoscopy, and you are unsure if you have endometriosis or not, allow a week off after your operation. This will suit most women. However, if you already know that you have endometriosis or if your endometriosis turns out to be severe you may need two weeks off, so don't plan your surgery before an important event. If you need any special bowel preparation before your surgery (see page 51), you may need the day before surgery off too. Some women bounce back quickly, even after major surgery, while others take longer. It is important to accept yourself and your needs whatever group you fit into. Recovering quickly does not make you a better person, just lucky.

Laparoscopies do make your abdomen sore, so you will need pain relief after your operation. Anything stronger than paracetamol or a period pain medication can make you constipated, so a high fibre diet, and a mild laxative are useful. A hot pack on your abdomen is comforting and relaxing. In my experience, women with chronic fatigue, chronic stress, or a lack of support at home, sometimes take longer to recover.

After your operation, you should gradually improve each day, but you will need more rest than normal. A daily walk is good exercise for your recovery, and it is safe to begin walking as soon as you leave hospital. Even a walk around your garden is a start. In general, if an activity hurts, don't do it, and if you are tired, have a rest. If you do too much on one day, you will be more tired the next day. If you are worried that you are not improving as quickly as you expected, ring your doctor. This is particularly important if you notice any of the following signs:

- A high temperature or fever. This can mean an infection.
- Pain in your leg. This can mean a clot in your leg veins.
- Difficulty breathing. This may mean a clot in your lungs or a lung condition such as pneumonia.
- Worsening nausea.
- Worsening pain.

Where does the gas go?

The gas used at a laparoscopy is called carbon dioxide (CO_2). This is the same gas that our bodies make as we turn the food we eat and the oxygen we breathe into energy, so it is a gas that our bodies are used to. CO_2 is breathed out through our lungs.

At the end of your laparoscopy most of the gas will be removed through the navel, but a small amount remains inside. *This gas is* around *the bowel* not *inside it*, so is absorbed by the body rather than passed as wind. This last bit of gas may cause shoulder pain if it lies near the diaphragm, because our brain feels any irritation of the diaphragm in the shoulder. Lying flat or even slightly head down allows the gas to float away from the diaphragm and the pain to improve. It should go away over a few days.

A laparoscopy to look for endometriosis needs to be very thorough. Endometriosis lesions may be subtle and can hide behind other pelvic organs. This means that some women who have had a laparoscopy with no abnormality found in the past, especially if it was more than five or ten years ago, may in fact have endometriosis now. It may have been in a form that was not recognised as endometriosis. This is not an error on the part of the gynaecologist, more a reflection of the lack of knowledge about endometriosis at that time. It is also possible that there truly was no endometriosis at the last laparoscopy but that it has formed since then.

Which endometriosis lesions cause pain – and what is 'awake laparoscopy'?

Not all lesions seen through a laparoscope are painful.

The question of which lesions hurt, and which do not, has

been investigated using *awake laparoscopy*. This means a laparoscopy done with local rather than general anaesthetic. The woman is given just enough sedation to be comfortable, but not asleep. She is awake enough to talk to her doctor during the operation and describe which parts of her pelvis are painful. The gynaecologist uses very delicate instruments to touch each area of the pelvis in turn. As each area is touched, the woman is asked whether she feels pain in that area and whether the pain she feels is the same as her normal pain. This process is called *pain mapping*.

A Canadian study using awake laparoscopy showed that not all endometriosis lesions were painful (see Reference 6). The lesions most likely to be painful were the red lesions or lesions with many blood vessels around them. The next most likely to be painful were the clear or white lesions, and the least likely to be painful were the black lesions. Only about one in four black lesions were painful to touch. They also found that touching normal-looking peritoneum up to 2 cm away from an endometriosis lesion might also cause pain in some women. Peritoneal windows (Chapter 1, page 8) were almost always painful.

Awake laparoscopies are *rare* operations and *never* done without the woman's consent.

How is a 'chocolate cyst' removed at a laparoscopy?

A chocolate cyst (endometrioma) has two parts: the cells around the edge of the cyst (the cyst wall) and the brown fluid inside. Draining the brown fluid from the cyst helps decide what sort of cyst it is, but won't remove the cyst wall. Unless the cyst wall is removed or destroyed, the cyst usually reforms quite quickly.

The cyst wall can be removed by 'stripping' it away from the ovary or 'cauterising' it with electrical or laser instruments. Even when this is done the cyst may still return, but it is much less likely than after drainage alone. The trick is to try and remove the cyst, while leaving as much of the normal ovary behind as possible.

In older women with completed families, removing the ovary may be a better option if the ovary is badly affected by endometriosis. This is rarely necessary in younger women.

Endometriomas are not cancers but they do mean that there is severe endometriosis present. Severe endometriosis like this, if left untreated, is likely to cause scarring and adhesions over time. Scarring and adhesions make surgery more difficult (see Chapter 9 on page 174).

Figure 5.2 An endometrioma

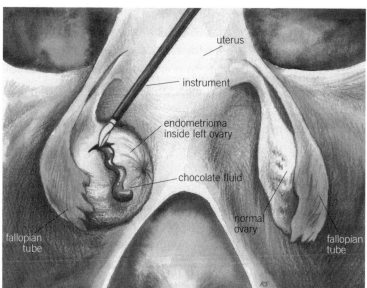

The left ovary is enlarged by an endometrioma (chocolate cyst). Opening the cyst releases a dark brown fluid. Once the cyst fluid and the cyst wall have been removed from inside the ovary, the ovary can return to normal size.

Could I need a larger cut for my surgery?

Sometimes a larger **incision** on the abdomen is necessary so that your endometriosis can be removed completely or for reasons of safety. Almost all endometriosis surgery can be done through small holes, so this is uncommon, but even the best endometriosis surgeons need to make a larger cut sometimes. As larger cuts take longer to heal, it is always a good idea to plan your surgery at least a few weeks before any important events – just in case.

If a larger cut is necessary, then the size and position of the cut will depend on what surgery is needed. Generally it will be either a cut across the lower part of the abdomen, similar to the scar from a caesarean birth, or a vertical cut from near the navel down to the pubic bone.

Do I need an operation?

Endometriosis is a surgical condition. This means that it is a condition where surgery plays a major role. Without a laparoscopy it cannot be reliably diagnosed, and for most women a laparoscopy with complete removal of their endometriosis is the treatment most likely to improve their symptoms for the longest period of time.

However, it is important to understand that the choice of whether or not to have an operation is always *yours*. Endometriosis is *not* a life-threatening condition. You will not die of endometriosis even if it feels like it.

The time to have an operation comes when the benefits *to you* of investigating your problems are greater than the risks *to you* of the operation. This is true of all surgery, but especially true of endometriosis surgery. So, faced with the choice of whether or not to have an operation, different women often make different choices.

However, by the time most women come to me they are ready for an operation. Their quality of life is poor. Other pain treatments have failed and they feel unable to continue as they are. Pain may have interrupted their employment, education or relationships.

The risks of surgery are small in comparison to a life of pain. A laparoscopy with removal of any endometriosis found is often a sensible choice. Even if complications occur, these women rarely regret their operation.

For other women, their pain is minimal. They have no fertility concerns and other treatments control their pain well. These women have less to gain from surgery and the decision whether or not to have a laparoscopy should be considered carefully. If there are complications during their operation these women are more likely to regret their decision.

Occasionally there are women with no symptoms at all but significant concerns who *choose* to have a laparoscopy. This group includes those with a family history of endometriosis who are concerned that they may be affected too, and wish to look after their pelvis for future fertility. A normal laparoscopy is reassuring for them, whereas finding endometriosis allows earlier and, it is hoped, more effective treatment.

Before deciding to have a laparoscopy, you should consider how significant your symptoms or other reasons are. If the following are all true, then a laparoscopy may be a good choice for you:

- Your symptoms are a problem to you, or you have good reason to suspect that you may have endometriosis
- You feel comfortable that you have enough information to decide
- You accept the uncommon but real risk of surgical complications, and
- Your gynaecologist will be able to remove any endometriosis found

> **If you have decided to have a laparoscopy, you should discuss with your surgeon what type of surgery you would like if endometriosis were found.**

For example, there are two possible options for treating a badly damaged ovary. Either the endometriosis can be removed and as much normal ovarian tissue as possible kept, *or,* the entire ovary can be removed together with its endometriosis. Both types of surgery are reasonable in different circumstances. The first option would suit a young woman, whereas an older woman with a completed family might choose to have the ovary removed and lessen the chance that she will need further surgery in the future (see Chapter 8, page 130).

Do laparoscopies cause scars?

Yes, but they are small and fade over time. How large the scars are, how many there are, and where they are, depends on how much surgery you need and your particular gynaecologist. Surgical techniques vary between different doctors, and the cuts are made in places that suit the surgical technique used.

Almost all laparoscopies start with a cut near the navel. This is usually easy to hide amongst the skin folds. Scars are red soon after the operation, but change to white over one or two years. A white scar will show more on tanned skin.

Keloid scars are a special type of scar. They are very thick, red and rise above the surface of the skin. Keloid scars are related to skin type, not the way a scar was stitched. They are more common in areas around the neck and in dark-skinned women.

How can I prepare for my laparoscopy?

Mental preparation

Having an operation can be daunting as it means giving control of your health to other people (your surgical team) for a period of time. While you are asleep, it is your surgical team who will make decisions for you. If you are someone who controls your life carefully (as many women do), you may find this idea hard to cope with. *However, the chance you won't wake up is virtually zero* and having thought through your options carefully (Chapter 4, page 46), you have a good reason for your surgery.

Anxiety before an operation is normal. If you are nervous, you may be able to visit the hospital before the day of your surgery. This allows you to become familiar with the hospital, and what will be done on the day. You may also wish to discuss a 'pre-med' with your anaesthetist. This medication will ease your anxiety when you go into theatre. The operation consent form should be signed before a pre-med is given, so plan ahead with your doctor. Pre-meds are not given to everyone as women wake up more quickly without them, and some laparoscopies are done as day surgery.

Remember that you are allowed to look forward to your surgery. Many women do. Sensibly they may be anxious about the risks involved, but the operation is a positive step they have chosen to improve their quality of life.

If possible, be kind to yourself in the days before your operation. With so many responsibilities, work commitments and dependents, many women work extra hard right up to the time of their surgery. They aim to have everyone and everything perfectly organised while they recover. Admirable though this may be, the overwork combined with normal anxiety before an operation means that they arrive in hospital stressed. Once the operation is over they collapse with exhaustion. This is similar to the headache that some overworked men or women get a few days into a holiday. Once the adrenalin stops pumping they fall in a heap. Your time spent in hospital and recovering at home may be the opportunity for your family to learn some useful life skills and take on more responsibility. They may be pleased to feel needed and repay the care you have given them over many years.

Smoking

Smoking is never a good idea and any time is a good time to quit. Before an operation is a particularly good time. As smoking is not permitted in hospitals and the urge to smoke is less after an anaesthetic, it is also an excellent time to make this change perma-nent. Smoking does not mean you can't have an operation, but it does increase the risk of serious lung infection (pneumonia) in the recovery period.

Frequently this is the first time that a smoker is confronted with the consequences of their smoking.

> ### I have a pierced navel. Will I need to remove my ring?
>
> Usually, yes. A ring might get in the way of the telescope, can increase the risk of a skin infection and because it is made of metal may not be safe near electrical instruments. While the risks of leaving it in are small, most surgeons will ask you to remove it. If you cannot remove the ring yourself, ask one of the nursing staff to remove it for you once you are asleep. The ring can be replaced at the end of your operation before you wake up.

Medications

Aspirin, or any medication that contains aspirin, should be stopped at least seven days before your surgery. This is because aspirin increases the risk of bleeding at your operation. Most period pain medications (see Chapter 6, page 63) are related to aspirin but can be continued until three or four days before surgery. Paracetamol and codeine medications are good choices for pain relief at this time because they do not increase the risk of bleeding.

If you are on medications that thin the blood such as *warfarin* or *heparin*, you should discuss this with your doctor and anaes-thetist at least two weeks before your operation.

If you are on the *contraceptive pill,* ask your doctor if this should be stopped before your operation. While being on the Pill does increase the risk of leg clots, the risk is still low in young women. Being on the Pill avoids the risk of an unplanned pregnancy, avoids difficulty timing the operation with the menstrual cycle and avoids even worse pain with periods.

Remember to tell your doctor about all the medications you are on, including those you can buy without a prescription, and any complementary therapies.

Bowel preparation

It is important to have an empty bowel during your surgery because:

- An empty bowel lies out of the way during the operation. This makes the operation easier for your gynaecologist to do and makes damage to the bowel less likely
- An empty bowel helps avoid constipation after your operation
- If a hole is made in your bowel, repair of the bowel is simpler and safer if the bowel is empty.

To empty the bowel your gynaecologist may recommend either a small enema or *bowel prep* before your operation, depending on what surgery is planned. The small enema empties the lower bowel, while bowel prep clears your entire bowel. From your surgeon's point of view, bowel prep is preferable, but as bowel prep is more trouble to you, they may reserve this for women where surgery near the bowel is expected. Bowel prep makes your surgery safer and easier.

What is the difference between a small enema and 'bowel prep'?

A small enema involves inserting a small amount of fluid (about 20 ml) just inside the anus, holding it inside for as long as possible (maybe 15 or 30 minutes) and then opening your bowels. It only clears the lower bowel.

Bowel prep involves two days of preparation before the day of your surgery. There are several types of bowel prep.

Older bowel prep medications such as Go-Lightly involved drinking four litres of medication. This was very difficult for women to do. Newer medications such as Picolax involve two drinks of about 100 ml each. This is much more acceptable. After the medication is taken, diarrhoea starts. How much diarrhoea there is depends a lot on how your bowel works normally. Women who are usually constipated may only open their bowels a few times, whereas women who tend to diarrhoea may have almost continual diarrhoea. Either way, it is advisable to be at home once you start the medication. You may need to open your bowels with little warning. It is important to drink a lot of water during this time.

Pregnancy

It is very *important that you are* not *pregnant at the time of your operation.* A laparoscopy during pregnancy might put your own health or the health of the baby at risk. If there is any chance you may be pregnant, tell your doctor. The date of your surgery may need to be altered, or a pregnancy test done. This is important, even if you would not choose to keep the pregnancy. Pregnancy tests are not reliable until at least the time of a missed period, so there is a window of time when no-one can tell if you are pregnant or not. Diagnosing pregnancy may also be difficult in women with irregular periods.

If you are currently trying to become pregnant, then you are unlikely to be using contraception. Your operation should be booked in the first half of your menstrual cycle after your period, but before ovulation has occurred (see Chapter 8, page 123). This is the time of the month when pregnancy is unlikely. If your periods are irregular or timing is difficult, ask your doctor about the best time for your surgery.

Back or joint conditions

Lying in one position on an operating table for prolonged periods of time sometimes aggravates a pre-existing back problem, or occasionally puts pressure on a nerve near the surface of the skin. Luckily, most women with back conditions find the position used at laparoscopy comfortable. If you do have any back or joint problems, you can ask to be positioned on the operating table while still awake. This allows you to ensure that your position is comfortable before going to sleep.

Other medical conditions and allergies

Any medical conditions such as diabetes or heart disease should be reported to your doctor and anaesthetist. If you have a family history of blood clots, easy bruising or bleeding, be sure to tell your doctor at least two weeks before the operation day. You may need special blood tests to make your operation safer.

Always tell your doctor if you have any *allergies*. A list of the medications that you are allergic to, as well as a list of those that you have taken in the past *without* problems is useful. Ultimately, you will need some medications during your stay in hospital, so knowing which medications do *not* cause you problems will help your doctor decide which medications to use.

What complications could there be?

Endometriosis surgery is difficult surgery. That is why not all gynaecologists do it. Apart from cancer surgery, it is the most difficult surgery we do. With this difficulty come some risks.

Every day throughout the world hundreds of laparoscopies are done. Only a very small number of these have major complications. However, although they are uncommon, complications from endometriosis surgery are particularly distressing. They occur in otherwise healthy young women.

> All surgery has risks that must be considered, but not having surgery has risks too. If you have endometriosis there is *no* option that has all benefits but no risks.

For most women, the risks of a laparoscopy can be divided into three groups:

- The general risks of an operation. These depend on your general health and how long the operation takes
- The risks involved in having a laparoscope and instruments inserted into your abdomen, and
- The risks involved with removing your endometriosis.

The general risks of an operation

These include:

- An allergic reaction to any medicines that are used
- A blood clot in the legs which may pass to the lungs
- Temporary aggravation of a previous back injury from lying in one position
- Breathing difficulties such as asthma or a lung infection (pneumonia) after your operation. This particularly applies to smokers.

The anaesthetist who puts you to sleep will stay with you throughout your operation. He or she monitors your heartbeat, breathing, temperature and position to make your operation as safe as possible.

The risks associated with inserting laparoscopic instruments and removing endometriosis

These risks may occur with *any* laparoscopy including a sterilisation operation to prevent pregnancy, removal of the appendix, or removal of the gall bladder. They can occur even in laparoscopies where no endometriosis is found. However, the more difficult the surgery is, the higher the risk.

These risks include:

1 Infection in a skin wound
2 A urine infection
3 Constipation or nausea after your operation
4 Shoulder tip pain (see Chapter 5, page 43) for a few days
5 Unintentional pressure on a nerve during an operation (a neuropathy). This pressure sometimes prevents the nerve from working normally for a period of time. Luckily, most neuropathies fully recover without treatment but they may take months to do so.
6 A hernia through one of the small cuts (one in 500 cases). This means a bulge near one of the small cuts. It can be repaired at a separate operation.
7 Adhesions from the surgery (see Chapter 9, page 174). Any surgery can cause adhesions, but they are less common after laparoscopic surgery than after surgery through larger cuts. Endometriosis itself can cause adhesions even without surgery.
8 An unintentional hole (perforation) in a blood vessel or pelvic organ (1 in 250 cases) (see Reference 7).

> **These lists include the most common and the most severe complications. They do not include every possible problem that could occur. If there are particular complications that you are anxious about, you should talk to your gynaecologist about them before your operation.**

What it means to have a perforation of an abdominal organ

This is the complication that worries both women and gynaecologists most. The organs involved might include the bladder, bowel, ureter, or some large blood vessels.

Not all perforations (holes) are a major problem, but some are. Whether or not they are a problem depends on whether the hole can be seen and repaired during the operation, and what type of surgery is needed to fix it.

Sometimes it is *necessary* to make a hole in the bowel or the bladder on purpose so that the endometriosis can be removed completely. Once the endometriosis is removed, the hole is repaired. This is good surgery rather than a complication. Without making the hole, some endometriosis would be left behind and your symptoms might not improve.

Even an *unintentional* hole in an organ may not be a serious problem. If it can be recognised and repaired at the time, and particularly if it can be done through the laparoscope, then although your recovery from surgery may be slower than planned, the long-term results are usually good.

Some of the most difficult cases are those where damage to an important organ, like ureter or bowel, was not recognised at the time of surgery. It may be that the hole was too small to see, or that the hole formed after the operation was finished. The electrical instruments used in most laparoscopic surgery may sometimes cause damage that does not show up until after the procedure is finished. During the operation, the damaged organ looks normal, but over the next few days, the damaged tissue breaks down and a hole forms. It is also possible for an infection in the pelvis to form an abscess that bursts, making a hole.

The effects of a perforated organ depend on which organ it is.

A hole in the bladder

A hole in the bladder can be repaired either through the laparoscope or through a larger cut. A soft rubber tube called a **catheter** is inserted into the bladder for between three and seven days after the operation to keep the bladder empty while it heals. The catheter drains urine into a bag over this time. The bladder heals well, and after the catheter is removed there are usually few problems.

A bladder perforation while dividing adhesions

Eleanor is a 60-year-old retired teacher in excellent health. Her past history included a hysterectomy for an enlarged uterus, and removal of her left ovary due to severe endometriosis many years ago. After some pain on the right side of her pelvis, an ultrasound showed a cyst on her right ovary. At 60 years of age, a cystic ovary could mean a cancer of the ovary. It was important to find out what the cyst was and to remove it.

At laparoscopy her pelvis was full of adhesions. Everything was stuck together. A thick curtain of fatty tissue blocked any view of the right side of her pelvis where the ovary would be. The adhesions were slowly and carefully divided so that the right ovary could be seen. However, during division of these adhesions a hole was made in the bladder. The bladder had been pulled up much higher than normal by the adhesions, and this unusual position had put it more at risk. After dividing all the adhesions, and removing what turned out to be a benign (not cancerous) ovarian cyst, the bladder was repaired through the laparoscope. A catheter was inserted to keep the bladder empty while it healed.

Eleanor stayed seven days in hospital instead of two, but was otherwise well. The catheter was removed after seven days, and she was able to pass urine normally. Although the hole in the bladder was unintended, no long-term damage resulted.

A hole in the bowel

If a hole in the bowel is recognised during an operation, it is repaired at the time. The technique used varies according to whether or not the bowel is empty, which part of the bowel is damaged, and the surgical skills available. The repair might be possible through the laparoscope, but a larger cut may be needed. Repair may be easier in women who have used 'bowel prep' before their surgery (see Chapter 5, page 51).

Sometimes a hole in the bowel forms after the operation is finished. Other holes may be too small to see at the time of the operation. The woman involved may look well after her surgery but become very ill later on, often after she has gone home. Her pain may increase, there may be vomiting and she may have a fever. This is an emergency situation requiring urgent medical attention. Repair of the hole usually requires a large cut on the abdomen, and may require a short-term **colostomy**. A colostomy means that the bowel empties into a bag outside the body on the abdominal wall. After three to six months, when the bowel has recovered, the colostomy is repaired at another operation. Once the bowel is rejoined, faeces can be passed normally again. This complication is a major problem for the woman involved, and her family. It is a complication that we, as surgeons, constantly try to avoid.

A bowel perforation with colostomy

Vivian is a 25-year-old married woman with one child. Her periods were painful and a laparoscopy found endometriosis that was removed. The pain improved, but two years later she returned unable to become pregnant and with painful periods once more. Laparoscopy showed more endometriosis, very close to the rectum (lower bowel), which was removed. Vivian was well the next day, but two weeks later suddenly became very unwell. Vivian had a hole in her bowel with infection throughout her abdomen (peritonitis). She went straight to surgery where a large cut on her abdomen was made. A small hole in the bowel next to where her surgery had been was found and repaired. However, a colostomy was needed in order to rest her bowel and allow the hole to heal. After four months the colostomy was closed at a separate operation and bowel actions emptied normally again. Vivian required major surgery, time in intensive care, and three months off work. No-one wishes to cause such a serious injury to another person. It has been a major problem for Vivian and her family.

A hole in a large blood vessel

There are several large blood vessels in and around the pelvis. They include the aorta, the inferior vena cava and the iliac blood vessels. Damage to one of these blood vessels, although very uncommon, is an emergency situation that usually requires a large cut in the abdomen to repair.

Damage to the ureter

The ureter is an important tube that passes from the kidney to the bladder on each side of the pelvis. The ureter lies in the side wall of the pelvis underneath the ovary. This is the most common place to find endometriosis, so removing endometriosis usually means operating very close to it. Any scar tissue present makes the ureter difficult to see and therefore difficult to avoid.

To make things even more difficult, some women are born with two ureters on one or both sides of their pelvis. Gynaecologists avoid damage to the ureter by finding it, and then staying as far away from it as possible. If there is a second, unknown ureter hidden amongst the endometriosis or scar tissue, then the second one may be damaged despite due care.

A damaged ureter may be very difficult to recognise during an operation. The woman involved may look and feel well after her surgery, but later develop pain in the loin area near the kidney on that side. An operation through a large cut is usually required to repair the ureter.

J have a large scar on my abdomen. Does that matter?

Yes. Women with an 'up-and-down' cut on their abdomen have a higher risk of bowel perforation at a laparoscopy. This is because a piece of bowel may have become stuck to the back of the scar during the healing phase of the previous operation. If so, then it is possible to make a hole in the bowel while the telescope is being inserted, before your doctor has a chance to see what is inside. A vertical scar does not mean that you cannot have a laparoscopy, but you should realise that there is an increased risk.

Does my general health affect the chance of a complication?

Yes, definitely. The two examples below illustrate the different risks among different women.

A healthy, normal weight, non-smoking 20-year-old woman, who has a laparoscopy where no abnormality is found, has the risks associated with having an anaesthetic as well as the risks involved in inserting instruments into the abdomen, but that is all. The risk for her of having an anaesthetic is very low. She is as likely to die driving her car to the hospital as die of the anaesthetic. The risk of a perforated organ as the instruments are inserted is small, but difficult to quantify. It may be approximately 1 in 500 laparoscopies. If endometriosis is found, then removing it will increase the risk, but also the possible benefits of her surgery.

A 45-year-old woman who has smoked for 20 years, is overweight, and has severe endometriosis, has higher anaesthetic, laparoscopy and endometriosis surgery risks to consider. The extra fatty tissue inside her abdomen restricts the view through the laparoscope and pushes the bowel closer to the instruments.

There is less room to work in her pelvis, and more chance of damage to the bowel. Her long-term smoking habit will make breathing difficulties such as asthma or pneumonia more likely after her surgery. Removing her endometriosis makes the operation longer and makes the chance of a hole in a pelvic organ greater. Smoking, middle age, overweight and a longer operation time all increase the chance of a blood clot in her legs. Even so, this woman has risks associated with surgery through a larger cut too, so if she truly does need an operation, a laparoscopy is still a good choice.

So why would any woman choose to have a laparoscopy?

They do so because their pain is severe, they are trying to become pregnant, or they suspect they have endometriosis. Surgery offers the only reliable diagnosis, and the most successful treatment for women with endometriosis.

> **Your surgeon's experience with endometriosis is very important, but all surgeons have complications at some time. In addition, those surgeons with the most experience are sent the most difficult cases requiring the most difficult surgery with the highest risk. There is _no_ surgeon who can promise that all will go well, but experience and good laparoscopic surgery skills do count.**

It is very reasonable for you to ask your particular surgeon what complications they have encountered before. Most will be quite open with this information, and welcome the opportunity to be frank about possible problems.

Chapter 6
. . . .

Which medicines are used to manage endometriosis?

THIS CHAPTER DESCRIBES the medications women with endometriosis often use or have recommended to them by their doctor. They are divided into:

- Anti-prostaglandin (period pain) medications (ibuprofen, naproxen, diclofenac etc)
- Pain killers (paracetamol, codeine, etc)
- GnRH analogues (leuprolide, triptorelin, nafarelin etc)
- Other medications to treat pain (amitriptyline, gabapentin, pregabalin)
- Progestogen medications (Mirena, Provera, norethisterone, etc)
- Contraceptive pill
- Danazol and gestrinone
- New treatments for endometriosis

> Whichever medicine you take, it is important to discuss possible side effects, other medications you already use, and any medical conditions you have with your doctor first. Only paracetamol and codeine are suitable for women who may be pregnant.

Anti-prostaglandin (period pain) medications (NSAIDs)

These medicines are also known as 'non-steroidal anti-inflammatory drugs', 'anti-inflammatory medications' or 'NSAIDs'. They include common period pain medications such as ibuprofen (Nurofen), naproxen (Naprogesic), diclofenac (Voltaren), indomethacin (Indocid) and mefenemic acid (Ponstan). They work by stopping your body making chemicals called prostaglandins.

Prostaglandins are very powerful chemicals that are made by the uterus around period time. They cause the crampy pain. It is prostaglandins that put a woman into labour when she has a baby, so it is not surprising that they can cause very severe pain. NSAID medications can help pain that is due to prostaglandins.

Whereas pain tablets like codeine work because they make the brain think it doesn't hurt, an NSAID works by treating the cause of the pain. By themselves they can treat mild or moderate pain, but when combined with other pain tablets such as codeine or paracetamol they can treat more severe pain.

Anti-prostaglandin medications are particularly useful as one part of the pain relief given after a laparoscopy. When tissues are irritated during surgery they make a lot of prostaglandins, which contribute to the pain. Even when stronger pain medications are needed, taking an NSAID as well gives a better quality of pain relief. They minimise the need for stronger pain medications

(opioids). It is the opioids that are most likely to cause nausea, vomiting and constipation.

Most NSAIDs are taken as tablets, but the strongest forms of NSAIDs come as suppositories. Suppositories are a medication mixed in a soft pellet made from cocoa butter or paraffin. They are pushed through the anus into the bowel and absorbed into the body through the bowel wall. They work well for period pain, and last for 12 hours, but I rarely have much luck suggesting them to teenagers!

NSAIDs should not be taken in pregnancy. They are also not suitable for women who are elderly, take blood pressure medications, have kidney disease, have stomach ulcers or stomach irritation, or whose asthma is triggered by aspirin-like medications.

How anti-prostaglandin medications work (see Fig 6.1)

Prostaglandins are made in the uterus from a substance called arachidonic acid. Arachidonic acid is present in the uterus all the time without causing pain, but at period time an enzyme called *cyclo-oxygenase (COX)* changes it into prostaglandins, and the pain starts.

NSAID medicines block the COX enzyme, and stop the uterus making prostaglandins from arachidonic acid. This is how they treat the pain and why it is important to take these medications either at the first sign of pain, or even before the pain starts. Once the prostaglandins have been made, an NSAID will not remove them. This is why they are much less effective when taken once the pain is severe. The individual NSAIDs vary, so you may find that one type of NSAID is more effective than others.

There are two types of cyclo-oxygenase (COX) enzyme, called COX-1 and COX-2. Normal anti-prostaglandin medications block both types, but some of the newer anti-prostaglandin medications only block COX-2. They are called 'COX-2 inhibitors' and include celecoxib (Celebrex) and lumiracoxib (Prexige).

COX-2 inhibitors still block the pain, because it is the COX-2 enzyme that is important for period pain. They seem to be less likely to cause stomach irritation than most anti-prostaglandin medications, but they have a higher risk of heart attack or stroke if used long term.

Figure 6.1 How anti-inflammatory medications work

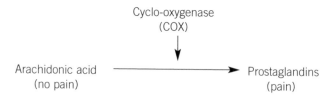

Anti-prostaglandin medications can prevent the COX enzyme making prostaglandins, but cannot remove them once they are made.

Pain killers

Paracetamol

Paracetamol is useful for mild to moderate pain, and is especially effective if taken together with an NSAID or codeine. It is important never to take more than eight of the 500 mg paracetamol tablets in one day, or liver damage may occur. If you use other tablets that have paracetamol in them, this paracetamol must be included in your total daily dose.

Opioid medications (also called narcotics)

Opioids were originally made from opium poppies. Some still are but others are made in laboratories. Opioid medications include codeine, oxycodone, tramadol, methadone, morphine, fentanyl and pethidine. The common opioids used by women at home include codeine, oxycodone, and tramadol. Pethidine, fentanyl and morphine are generally only used in hospitals.

All opioid medications can cause constipation and nausea but some women are more sensitive to these effects than others.

Codeine is a 'pro-drug'. This means it must be converted into another drug by our body to have the best effect. Codeine itself has some effect on pain but it is much more effective when converted by the body into morphine. To change codeine into morphine requires an enzyme called CYP2D6. As some people don't have this enzyme, some people don't find codeine very useful for their pain. They get a benefit from the codeine itself, but not the morphine benefit that others receive. Codeine is usually prescribed in doses of 8 to 60 mg every three to four hours. It is often combined in a tablet with either paracetamol or aspirin.

Figure 6.2 How codeine is converted to morphine

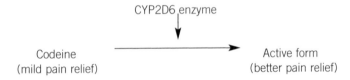

Women whose bodies do not make the CYP2D6 enzyme will find codeine less helpful for their pain than other women.

Oxycodone is a strong opioid medication that can be taken as a tablet. It has a similar effect to morphine. Oxycodone can be taken as slow release tablets that work for a longer period of time. This means that they do not need to be taken as often.

Tramadol is a medication for pain with a mixture of actions. Tramadol has a weak opioid effect (like codeine), but more importantly it affects a chemical in the brain called serotonin. Tramadol may be useful for moderate pain but is not strong enough for severe pain. It is quite a complicated medication and can cause side effects that include nausea, dizziness, vomiting, confusion and occasionally epileptic fits. It should be avoided by women with epilepsy and used with care in women who take any of the following medications or herbal preparations:

• Tricyclic medications (this includes amitriptyline)

- St John's wort
- Ondansetron (an anti-nausea medication)
- A group of medications called selective serotonin reuptake inhibitors (SSRIs). These are used to treat depression and anxiety.

GnRH analogues

There are many different GnRH analogues. The commonly used ones include leuprolide (Prostap), triptorelin (Decapeptyl), nafarelin (Synarel) and goserelin (Zoladex).

Natural GnRH is a hormone made by the brain. It tells the ovary to prepare an egg for ovulation and make the hormone oestrogen. GnRH analogue medications look like natural GnRH to our bodies, but act differently. They stop natural GnRH from working and block the message from the brain to the ovary. An egg is not released and very little oestrogen is made. Oestrogen levels become very low indeed: much lower than with danazol or gestrinone. Androgen (testosterone) levels are approximately normal.

The acid in our stomach would destroy GnRH analogues taken as tablets, so they are given either as a nasal spray twice a day (Synarel) or a long-acting injection once a month (Decapeptyl, Prostap or Zoladex). Treatment is started during a period and must *not* be used if you may be pregnant. There is a possible risk of miscarriage or birth abnormality if used during pregnancy.

The side effects of GnRH analogues are similar to a normal menopause, so while taking these medications, you and your mother may have more things in common than usual! The low oestrogen levels mean no periods, hot flushes, tiredness, night sweats, vaginal dryness, headaches, muscle pains, low libido and a tendency to thinning of the bones.

To manage these symptoms while on the treatment, many women take hormone replacement therapy. This contains oestrogen and progestogen, the two female hormones. When used with a GnRH analogue, this is called 'add-back therapy' and does not prevent its effect on endometriosis. While on this treatment it is a good idea to increase the calcium in your diet, or take a calcium tablet each day. This gives even more protection to your bones. It has been common for 'add-back therapy' to be given only after a month of GnRH analogue treatment alone. However, it has recently been shown that starting 'add-back therapy' from the beginning of GnRH analogue treatment is just as effective (See Reference 9).

Although there have been some concerns about the safety of long-term HRT in women after menopause, there are no concerns over the safety of HRT in women before menopause who are on a GnRH analogue. All doctors agree that it is a good idea. The HRT is only giving back a small amount of the hormone that the GnRH analogue has taken away. It is not providing extra hormone above the woman's normal levels. Once the GnRH analogue and add-back therapy cease, oestrogen levels return to normal and periods return.

Doctors disagree on how useful these medications are at treating endometriosis. Those gynaecologists who are experienced at removing endometriosis usually prefer excision surgery first and leave these medications for situations when surgery is not enough. Those gynaecologists who are less comfortable with endometriosis surgery usually diagnose endometriosis at a laparoscopy, and then recommend a course of medication. They keep further surgery for those women in whom medications have failed.

What all doctors agree is that there are *no* medicines (or herbal preparations) that are always effective, always safe, have no side effects, have no long term risks, are cheap to provide and easily available. If such a treatment existed, no one would recommend anything else.

The *advantage* of treating endometriosis with a GnRH analogue, rather than excising it at a laparoscopy is that it avoids *some* of the risks of an operation. It won't allow you to avoid an operation altogether because a laparoscopy is still needed to diagnose endometriosis in the first place. However, a laparoscopy that looks for endometriosis but does not remove it is shorter, safer and easier than a laparoscopy that looks for and removes endometriosis. My concern is that it is also less effective at managing pain.

The *disadvantages* of using a GnRH analogue include its side effects, the need to avoid pregnancy while taking the medication, the cost involved, and the fact that endometriosis symptoms often return once the medication is stopped. These medications rarely remove endometriosis. They suppress it.

What can I expect from a GnRH analogue?

Periods usually stop on these medications, so they are very good at treating period pain. They are less successful (but often still very good) at treating pelvic pain between periods, painful intercourse, or bowel pain, probably because women with these symptoms usually have some scar tissue present.

> **GnRH analogues will not remove scar tissue, divide adhesions, remove chocolate cysts from an ovary or improve fertility. They work best on thin, small lesions.**

The biggest problem with their use is that pain often returns once the treatment stops. Any endometriosis that remains becomes active again, and the pain returns, often within about six months of stopping the medication. Even so, GnRH analogues can offer a welcome break from pain. They are also useful where some endometriosis (but not scar tissue) remains after surgery, or where surgery to remove endometriosis is unavailable.

Most GnRH analogues are given as a six-month course. Once the course is finished, many women start the contraceptive pill, used continuously, to try and maintain any benefits they have achieved. Alternatively, the end of a GnRH analogue course is a good time to have a Mirena IUD inserted. This decreases the chance that period pain will return.

Some women feel really well with low oestrogen levels. Those who have suffered hormone-related symptoms such as migraines during periods, or hormonal moodiness, sometimes really enjoy their time on GnRH analogues. Their hormonal cycle has been turned off, at least for six months, and they feel the best of their adult life. These women later find menopause a blessed relief.

GnRH analogue treatment and pain

Janine is a 37-year-old office worker. Over the last year she had noticed a severe pain just under her right rib cage with each period. It had taken a while for her to realise that this pain only happened on the first day of her period. Janine also had stress at work. Her boss was difficult and she was working long hours. A laparoscopy showed small areas of endometriosis in her pelvis, which were removed. No endometriosis was seen on the diaphragm, but as the liver hides part of the diaphragm, endometriosis at that site could not be completely excluded. Janine started Zoladex injections monthly for six months. During this time she had no periods and no right-sided pain. At the end of six months' treatment, Janine started the contraceptive pill taken continuously hoping to maintain the benefit achieved with the GnRH analogue medication. Periods were planned every three to four months. Janine also changed her job, became less stressed, and worked on her general health. There have been no further episodes of pain.

Endometriosis of the diaphragm is rare. To remove it may require major chest surgery. We may never know if it was present or not. However, the fact that the pain only happened with periods and that using the GnRH analogue to stop periods also stopped the pain, certainly suggests that the pain might be due to endometriosis. While her pain can be avoided with the contraceptive pill used continuously, there is no need for further treatment.

What about long term GnRH analogues and HRT without a laparoscopy?

In some countries, some doctors use GnRH analogues with 'add-back' HRT long-term for women with pelvic pain, without first doing a laparoscopy. They are never sure whether or not their patients actually have endometriosis, but it is presumed that they do. This form of treatment is used where a laparoscopy is considered too expensive to offer, or the skills to remove endometriosis surgically and safely are not available. It is not a treatment plan that I use, but may be reasonable in some cases.

My concerns are that:

- Some women without endometriosis will be treated unnecessarily
- Other causes of pelvic pain may be missed
- The treatment will not improve fertility
- This treatment is unlikely to remove large or deep areas of endometriosis

- Some women may have side effects from the medication
- Rarely, a cancer of the ovary could be missed.

Other medications to treat pain

Amitriptyline

Amitriptyline does not treat endometriosis, nor is it a normal painkiller, but it *is* very useful for women with pelvic pain. Amitriptyline helps women with pelvic pain in many ways:

- It treats 'neuropathic pain' (see Chapter 9, page 177), where the nerves from the pelvis to the brain have changed their structure and become sensitised. They send too many pain signals to the brain, which makes any pelvic pain feel even worse than it is. Neuropathic pain is very common in women with endometriosis, particularly those who have pain on most days of the month
- It helps pain from an irritable or painful bladder
- It can slow an irritable bowel
- It helps women who sleep poorly, because they have pain or they need to empty their bladder frequently
- It makes the pain after a laparoscopy easier to manage.

With so many possible benefits, it is not surprising that many women with chronic pelvic pain improve on amitriptyline. It rarely cures pain completely, but is a valuable part of the whole treatment plan.

The common side effects of amitriptyline include dry eyes, dry mouth, mild constipation, and drowsiness. However these side effects go away as your body becomes used to the medication. Starting with a small dose taken *at night* avoids most side effects and allows most women to use amitriptyline if they choose to. Even if you have tried amitriptyline before and felt unwell, you may still be able to use it if you start with a low dose, and increase the dose slowly.

There are many different treatment plans, but 5 mg at night is a good dose to start on. This is half a 10 mg tablet. This dose may not be enough to improve the pain but it is usually not enough to cause many side effects either. If you feel well and alert the next day, then the dose can be increased by 5 mg every few days until either your pain has improved or you reach 25 mg. If you feel at all sleepy, or your eyes or mouth are too dry then stay on the same dose each night until your body adjusts to the tablets. This might take a few days or a week. There is no rush: it is more important to feel well and avoid problems.

Very few women need more than 25 mg, so if you have reached this dose without any benefit, then amitriptyline may not be effective for you. If your pain improves at a dose lower than 25 mg, then stay on that dose. Many women find that 10 mg at night is all they need. Chewing gum or extra drinks help a dry mouth.

Amitriptyline is taken at night because it can cause drowsiness. This could be dangerous if you are driving a car or operating machines. If taken at night, then drowsiness is more of a benefit than a problem. Just in case it does make you sleepy, it is important to start it the evening before a quiet day when you do not need to drive a car or operate machines, until you can tell how you will feel. Amitriptyline does not mix well with alcohol. Any alcohol you do drink will affect you more than usual, so be careful!

Amitriptyline is not a medication to take every now and then. If you do start it, make the commitment to take it every night. Then consider whether it has helped. Amitriptyline is unlikely to completely resolve your pain, but are you better? Is your sleep better? Is your pain easier to manage? If so, then the amitriptyline should be continued for three to six months, or even longer. When you decide to stop it, decrease the dose slowly by 5 mg every few days, just as you did at the start. Do not stop it suddenly.

Amitriptyline is one of a group of drugs called 'tricyclics'. In the past, tricyclics were used in high doses (maybe 150 mg) to treat depression. If your doctor recommends amitriptyline, or a similar medication, it is not because they think your pain is psychological, or that you are depressed. They have recommended it for good medical reasons. Amitriptyline is no longer used to treat depression, because there are better drugs available. It is used in small doses to manage pain, an irritable bladder, an irritable bowel, or interrupted sleep.

Unlike a completely *un*related group of drugs called benzodiazepines, problems with addiction to tricyclics are uncommon. Benzodiazepines include drugs such as diazepam (Valium) or oxazepam (Serepax). These have very little place in the management of chronic pain, apart from muscle spasm.

> **There are some medical conditions, and some medications, that do not mix well with amitriptyline. This is why it is important that you talk to your doctor before starting it, and don't take it if you may be pregnant.**

Pregabalin and Gabapentin

These are new medications that help many women with chronic pain, especially those with pain that is aching, stabbing, sharp or burning. They affect how nerves send pain signals. (See Chapter 9, page 146)

A full dose of pregabalin is 75 mg twice daily, but to avoid the dizziness that can happen when starting the medication, it is best to start with a lower dose. I suggest that you start by cutting open and dissolving a 75 mg capsule in water or cordial. Drink half the water at night and half the next night. Continue with half a capsule each night until any dizziness has settled, then increase the dose to a whole 75 mg capsule each night. You will know within a few weeks if this medication will help your pain.

The side effects include dizziness, sleepiness, swollen ankles, impaired memory, bowel disturbances and the possibility of mild weight gain. Dizziness may be worse if you are also taking opioid medication such as oxycodone, or medications to treat anxiety such as lorazepam.

Progestogen medications (Mirena, norethisterone, medroxyprogesterone acetate)

Women with endometriosis use progestogen medications partly because they can delay periods and stop ovulation, but also because they make endometriosis lesions less active.

Progestogen medications are not the same as *Progesterone.* Progesterone is the hormone made by the ovary in the second half of the menstrual cycle after ovulation. A tablet of progesterone would be destroyed by the acid in the stomach, so synthetic versions of progesterone (progestogens) have been developed which survive in the stomach, and act like progesterone in the body.

The commonly used progestogen tablets include norethisterone (Primolut), medroxyprogesterone acetate (Provera), levonorgestrel (Microval), dydrogesterone (Duphaston) etonorgestrel (Implanon) and depot medroxyprogesterone acetate (Depo-Provera).

Many women take progestogens without any difficulty, but others find progestogen side effects unacceptable. Once again, we are all different.

The commonest side effect is 'break-through bleeding', which means vaginal bleeding at irregular and unpredictable times. This may be quite troublesome. Other side effects include moodiness, bloating, and headaches. Women who are 'progestogen sensitive' describe this feeling as being 'constantly premenstrual'.

When taken every day (continuously) progestogens stop periods, at least in most women, and avoiding periods means less period pain.

If you feel well on the contraceptive pill, you are unlikely to have many side effects with a progestogen medication.

A progestogen used to prevent period pain

Jane is a 43-year-old mother of three children. Five years ago, a laparoscopy performed to investigate her painful periods found endometriosis. Apart from severe pain during her period she was well. Jane started a progestogen medication taken every day and continued it for five years. Over this time she had no periods and no pain. Some women feel moody on progestogens, but Jane felt healthy and was happy that she could avoid the pain.

After five years, Jane noticed vaginal bleeding at odd times that became very persistent. An ultrasound showed a normal uterus with a very thin lining. The normal balance between oestrogen (which makes the lining thicker), and progesterone (which makes the lining thinner) had been disturbed. On her tablets Jane had more progestogen than oestrogen, and the lining of the uterus had become so thin that it bled easily, much like the thin skin on an old person's hands if they are knocked. There was nothing dangerous about a thin lining but the bleeding was annoying and unlikely to stop until the lining of the uterus became thicker and less delicate.

Jane stopped her progestogen tablets. Her oestrogen levels increased, the bleeding stopped and her periods returned. Unfortunately with the return of her periods came the period pain she had avoided for five years.

Figure 6.3 A Mirena IUD diagram

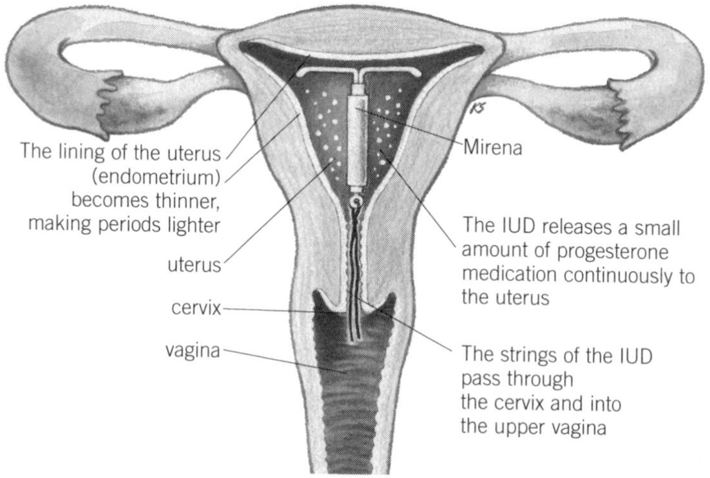

The lining of the uterus
(endometrium)
becomes thinner,
making periods lighter

Mirena

The IUD releases a small
amount of progesterone
medication continuously to
the uterus

uterus

cervix

vagina

The strings of the IUD
pass through
the cervix and into
the upper vagina

A levonorgestrel-releasing intra-uterine device (Mirena).

A progestogen-releasing intra-uterine device (Mirena)

Progestogen medications work well at avoiding periods and decreasing pain, so why are progestogen tablets, implants and injections unpopular? They are unpopular because many women just don't like the way that progestogens make them feel.

Most of these side effects can be avoided by attaching some progestogen medication to an intra-uterine device and inserting it into the uterus. (See Fig 6.3) This treats the pelvis with progestogen, but only a small amount of the progestogen reaches the rest of the body. The device is called a Mirena IUD and the progestogen medication it contains is called levonorgestrel.

Yes, you *can* use a Mirena for contraception, just like any IUD, but its particular benefit is to lighten periods, and often make them less painful.

An Italian study (see Reference number 12) looked at whether or not inserting a Mirena during a laparoscopy to remove endometriosis would give women longer lasting and better relief for their period pain. A year after their laparoscopy, 45 per cent of the women who just had a laparoscopy had bad period pain, whereas only 10 per cent of the women who had a laparoscopy *and* a Mirena had bad period pain.

If you plan to have a Mirena inserted, it is important to realise that irregular and annoying bleeding is quite common in the first three months after it is inserted. Not everyone gets this, but many women do. Once it settles, there is a good chance that you will have very little bleeding and hopefully less pain. Around 30 per cent of women have no periods at all with a Mirena IUD in place.

It is also common to have crampy pains after it is inserted. These pains usually settle within a few weeks but they can be severe. They are best treated with period pain medications (see Chapter 6, page 72). If you have been on the contraceptive pill, then continuing this for a month after your Mirena is inserted might minimise these problems.

When the IUD is inserted, there is a small chance that a pelvic infection may occur. Over time, such an infection may cause pain (see Chapter 9, page 204) or possibly block the fallopian tubes causing difficulty becoming pregnant. If you are considering having an IUD, talk to your doctor about your individual risk of infection and how an infection can be avoided. This will help you decide whether having an IUD is a good choice for you.

If you like the Mirena, it can stay in place and remain effective for five years. It can then be removed or replaced. If you don't like it for any reason, your doctor can remove it by pulling the strings that pass out through the cervix into your vagina.

In Japan, an IUD that releases a small amount of danazol to the uterus, rather than a progestogen has been used.

The contraceptive pill

The contraceptive pill should really be called a 'hormone management pill'. It has many uses apart from contraception, and is used by many women who are not sexually active and have no need for contraception. In women with endometriosis, it is particularly useful because:

- *The Pill is a good treatment for prostaglandin pain.* Prostaglandin pain is a major part of most period pain, but particularly in women who have not had children. It is also a part (but not all) of endometriosis pain. The Pill prevents ovulation. Blocking ovulation means less prostaglandins and less pain.
- *The Pill can be used 'continuously' to decrease the number of periods per year.* Fewer periods means less period pain. The Pill can also allow periods to be timed to avoid important events like exams or holidays. See page 80.
- *The Pill may prevent endometriosis in some women.* An Australian study found that women who had used the Pill for more than five years had a 30 per cent lower risk of endometriosis (see Reference number 10).

Newspapers and popular magazines frequently report negative things about the Pill but there are some positives too. Women on the Pill have less period pain, lighter periods, less ovulation pain, less premenstrual tension, more regular periods, fewer pimples and a lower risk of developing cancer of the ovary or uterus. It also provides good contraception.

Although the side effects of the Pill as they apply to you need to be carefully considered with your doctor, women with endometriosis may have a lot to gain from being on it.

How to use the Pill continuously (skipping periods)

Most women who use the Pill continuously still have periods, but their periods are two, three or four months apart rather than one month apart. They time their periods to fit their lifestyle.

If you wish to do this, you will need to use a 'monophasic' contraceptive pill. Monophasic pills have two different coloured tablets in each packet. There is one colour for the hormone tablets, and one for the inactive or 'sugar' tablets. 'Triphasic' pills have four different coloured tablets in the packet. They are not suitable for continuous use as troublesome bleeding usually occurs.

You should take a hormone tablet every day, with no sugar tablets until you plan a period. When you want to have a period, stop the hormone tablets for seven days, have a period and then restart the hormone tablets again.

If you want to have the longest possible time between periods, take a hormone tablet reliably every day, and wait until bleeding starts by itself. Some women can take the pill for six months without bleeding, whereas others bleed after only six weeks. Almost all women will start bleeding eventually.

Once you start bleeding, you should stop the Pill for seven days and have a period. You don't have to do this straight away if you are busy, but until you do have a period the bleeding will probably continue. The bleeding that happens on the hormone tablets is bleeding from the lining of the uterus. It does not take the place of a normal period.

After seven days off the hormone tablets, you should start them again and continue them until either you start to bleed or you choose to have a period. Provided that the hormone tablets are taken for at least 21 days between periods, and there is no more than seven days break between hormone tablets, you are no more likely to become pregnant than women using the Pill with monthly periods.

If you have a special event in mind and want to avoid having a period, it is safest to plan a period a couple of weeks before the event, so that it is unlikely you will be bleeding on the day. With seven days off the Pill, and then another week or so to settle, you will hopefully be pain and bleeding free at the chosen time. Students sometimes choose to have periods only during their holiday breaks. Other women might choose to have the worst days of their period on a weekend. Remember that if you miss any pills this tells the uterus to start a period, and you may bleed or have pain.

Is it dangerous to use the Pill continuously?

Despite the fact that many women skip periods with the Pill, there has been very little research into this question. If you take the Pill continuously for a whole year without any breaks, then you will have taken an extra three months of tablets during the year. This means that if there are any extra risks, they could be due to a higher hormone dose.

However, almost all the information we have on the Pill and its risks, is based on old studies that used pills with 35 to 50 mcg of oestrogen in each tablet. As the newer pills have only 20-30 mcg of oestrogen in each tablet, even if extra pills are taken, the total dose for the year is still less than the dose on which our current understanding of risk is based.

It is likely that we will soon have 15 mcg pills that are designed for a period every three months. These will provide an even lower total hormone dose than currently possible.

Using the Pill continuously provides *more* reliable contraception than the same pill used with a monthly period.

Endometriosis, prostaglandin pain and premenstrual syndrome

Jackie is a nurse aged 21 who suffered pelvic pain on most days of her cycle, but particularly with periods. Premenstrual syndrome (PMS) before her period was straining the otherwise good relationship she had with her family and boyfriend. A laparoscopy showed widespread endometriosis that was completely removed. At review a few months later the pain through the month had gone. This pain had been due to her endometriosis.

The first day of her period was still painful and she still had PMS. Jackie had worked hard at her general fitness and stress management. She felt better able to cope with her premenstrual symptoms and was generally healthier but still moody. Adding the contraceptive pill helped her PMS further, improved the prostaglandin period pain, provided contraception, and allowed her to skip periods. Over time it might provide some protection against further endometriosis. Jackie knows that at her age new areas of endometriosis may develop. However she feels comfortable knowing that if her pains recur then treatment is available.

Danazol and gestrinone

Danazol and gestrinone were commonly prescribed for endometriosis in the 1980s. They are less commonly used now, but do suit some women. Like GnRH analogues, they suppress endometriosis rather than remove it, and work best for women with thin, mild lesions.

Danazol and gestrinone work by making *oestrogen levels lower* and *androgen (testosterone) levels higher*.

Their side effects include:

- *Side effects due to higher androgen levels.* These include weight gain, slightly bulkier muscles, oily skin, increased body hair and cramps
- *Side effects due to low oestrogen levels.* These include lower libido (interest in sex), smaller breasts, and sometimes hot flushes.

Occasionally, there is a deepening of the voice. This is not a common side effect, but unlike the other side effects that go away once the danazol or gestrinone is stopped, a deeper voice may be irreversible. So, if you are a keen singer the small risk of a deeper voice is not worth taking and these medications are not for you.

Danazol is a banned substance for competitive athletes because it increases muscle strength. It may also affect blood sugar levels so should be used with care by women with diabetes.

It is very important *not* to become pregnant on danazol or gestrinone. If taken during pregnancy, it may cause abnormalities of the baby's genital organs.

Danazol is taken at a dose of 600 to 800 mg daily. Gestrinone capsules are taken at doses of 2.5 to 5 mg twice a week. Both medications are usually prescribed for six months. They are not used long term because their effect on blood fats might increase the risk of heart and blood vessel disease later in life. These risks are small when used for six months.

It is estimated that pain returns in 50 per cent of women within 12 months of stopping treatment. If the endometriosis is severe, then symptoms are even more likely to return (see Reference number 8). To try and maintain the benefits achieved, some women choose to start the contraceptive pill, taken continuously, (see Chapter 6, page 80) or have a Mirena IUD inserted at the end of their course of treatment.

> ## Danazol, gestrinone or a GnRH analogue. Which one is best for me?
>
> Your choice depends on which side effects you are least concerned about and what other problems you may have. For example, danazol and gestrinone make skin oiler and periods lighter. They are a good choice if you have heavy periods, but a poor choice if you have acne. GnRH analogues stop the menstrual cycle but also lower bone density. They are a good choice if you suffer premenstrual tension or severe headaches with periods (menstrual migraines), but a poor choice if you have thin bones. In general, GnRH analogues are better tolerated than danazol or gestrinone especially if 'add-back therapy' is used.

Other medications

Research into new medications continues. Several types of medications have been suggested, and if your endometriosis has been difficult to manage it is possible that one of these medications might be recommended to you. None of these new medications have been used by enough women for us to know how useful they are, nor what their side effects are. Their use is experimental and generally reserved for those women where more usual treatments have failed. They include:

- Aromatase inhibitors such as anastrozole and letrozole (see page 85)
- Hydroxychloroquine or methotrexate in women where 'inflammatory changes' are found at laparoscopy. (See page 207)
- Anti-oestrogen medications, such as tamoxifen or raloxifene
- Anti-tumour necrosis factor (anti-TNF) medications like infliximab

- Medications to discourage new blood vessel formation such as endostatin and TNP-470
- Medications that affect chemicals called matrix metalloproteinases
- Medications that affect immunity such as pentoxifylline.

How do aromatase inhibitors work?

Endometriosis lesions need oestrogen to survive. Some of the oestrogen they need comes from the ovaries but some is made in the endometriosis lesion itself.

The endometriosis lesion does this using an enzyme called aromatase that can convert other hormones into oestrogen. An endometriosis lesion likes lots of oestrogen and by making its own supply it is able to adapt its environment and promote its own growth. Having the enzyme aromatase also means that an endometriosis lesion can make its own supply of oestrogen even after both ovaries have been removed.

As the name suggests, aromatase inhibitors block aromatase and stop the endometriosis lesions from making their own oestrogen. In a woman who is through menopause and no longer makes oestrogen in her ovaries, this takes away the last supply of oestrogen available to an endometriosis lesion.

The major side effects of aromatase inhibitors are bone thinning, tiredness and menopausal symptoms, but there are others. These medications are usually only recommended for women after menopause, but have recently been used in women before menopause too.

Before considering this medication it is important that you understand the possible side effects and discuss them carefully with your doctor. They should never be taken during pregnancy.

Post-menopausal endometriosis treated with an aromatase inhibitor

The first gynaecologist to report using an aromatase inhibitor to treat endometriosis was a Japanese gynaecologist called Dr Takayama in 1998. (see Reference number 11). Dr Takayama treated a 57-year-old woman whose endometriosis had returned even after a hysterectomy, removal of both ovaries, and two extra operations for endometriosis blocking her ureter. Even after this surgery the woman returned with a painful 3 cm endometriosis lesion in the vagina. Because it was in the vagina, the lesion could easily be seen at vaginal examination. Dr Takayama could measure the size of the lesion before and after different treatments to see which treatment was most effective.

Four months of a progestogen medication did not help. The lesion stayed the same size and her pain continued. However within two months of starting anastrozole (an aromatase inhibitor), the pain had gone. After nine months of treatment the 3 cm lesion had shrunk to 3 mm. To try and minimise bone thinning while on the medication she was given calcium tablets and a medication called alendronate, which encourages bone formation. Even so, she lost six per cent of her bone density over the treatment period. There were no other side effects reported in her case.

Newer aromatase inhibitors in the future may be able to avoid bone thinning.

Chapter 7

Js this your situation?

FACTS ABOUT ENDOMETRIOSIS are one thing, but the most important question is *'What choices do I have now to manage my pain?'* Every woman's situation is different, but this is the question I have tried to answer in this chapter. You may find that one of these sections describes your situation.

The group left out are all the women whose endometriosis has been treated successfully by whatever method they chose. Not surprisingly, most of these women would prefer to forget about endometriosis and get on with their lives.

I am a teenager with severe period pain

Most teenagers have period pain of some sort. For most, this pain is due to chemical substances called prostaglandins that are made by the uterus at period time. Prostaglandin pain is usually quite easy to diagnose. It comes on the first day of bleeding, may be severe, but generally goes away with the Pill, or normal period pain medications if they are taken correctly. A teenager with prostaglandin pain may look quite sick on the first day of her period, yet be fully recovered only a few hours later. This is the pain that is rather unkindly called 'Normal period pain'. It is called 'normal' because the pelvis looks normal at a laparoscopy, *not because it doesn't hurt.* It does.

If you are a teenager, then you will have at least *some* prostaglandin pain, but if your pain doesn't fit the normal picture you may have endometriosis too. You may have worked out already that your pain is different to the other girls'. Your friends may argue (very reasonably) that there is nothing 'normal' about their pain, but it is probably not as bad as your pain.

None of us know what another woman's pain is like, but if your pain is *un*-manageable despite the Pill, or period pain medications, then consider endometriosis. It becomes even more likely if you have pain leading up to a period, pain like period pain at other times of the month, severe back pain, pain felt in one spot rather than generally across your abdomen, or pain opening your bowels. Your particular symptoms will depend on where the endometriosis is, so you may not have all these symptoms.

Severe period pain in young women is a bigger problem now than it was in the past. Our grandmothers often had their first baby before they were 20 years old. After that came years spent pregnant or breast-feeding until menopause arrived. Even if their periods were painful, at least they didn't have many of them. Our grandmothers probably averaged about 30 or 40 periods in a lifetime. Prostaglandin pain usually improves after having a baby, so one cause of their pain got better, even if their endometriosis remained.

Girls start their periods earlier now. They delay their first pregnancy and have fewer (if any) children. By 14 years of age, many have had periods for three or four years. They are still girls, but physically they are women. They may have 300 or 400 periods before menopause.

In the past, endometriosis was thought to be rare in teenagers. This is not true. An American study of teenagers with severe period pain, who were no better after trying medications, found that 70 per cent of them had endometriosis (Reference 14). If you have periods, you are *not* too young to have endometriosis.

> **If you are a young woman who has not had a baby, then some of your pain will be prostaglandin pain from the uterus. So, the question to ask is: 'Do I have prostaglandin pain with an otherwise healthy pelvis, or do I have both prostaglandin pain AND endometriosis causing my pain?'**

If you can manage your pain well with the Pill, a period pain medication or both, then your chance of having endometriosis is low. So, if there are no other reasons to suspect endometriosis, then a laparoscopy is probably not necessary. However, if medications don't help and your pain persists then it is time to talk to your general practitioner or a gynaecologist.

If you do have a laparoscopy and endometriosis is removed, this does not mean you will have no pain. You are still a young woman who has not had a child, so you will still have prostaglandin pain from your uterus. Removing endometriosis can only help symptoms that are due to endometriosis. What is hoped is that you will have *less* pain and that the pain you have will be easier to manage.

What can I do if my endometriosis has been removed but the first one or two days of my period are still very painful?

This period pain is coming from your uterus. In the old days, you would be advised to have your children quickly then have a hysterectomy. Nowadays, you can almost always manage the pain well with one or more of the following options.

- The contraceptive pill used continuously to cut down the

number of periods so you suffer pain less often (Chapter 6, page 80)

- Anti-inflammatory suppositories (Chapter 6, page 64) which seem to work better than anti-inflammatory tablets
- Continuous progestogen medicine to stop periods, either as tablets, a three-monthly injection, or a three-year implant (Chapter 6, page 75).
- A levonorgestrel intrauterine device (Chapter 6, page 77). This is a newer treatment, but worth considering.
- Vitamin E – 200 mg of natural vitamin E taken twice daily from two days before a period and for the first three days of a period
- Acupuncture
- Working to improve your health and fitness generally – this is always worthwhile. Healthy, happy people have less pain.

A teenager with period pain

Rosetta is a 16-year-old woman who came to see me with several problems. Rosetta had severe period pain for a week before and throughout her period. A similar milder pain bothered her at other times of the month without warning. She noticed spots of blood in her pants at odd times, but especially in the week before a period. Her worst day by far was the first day of her period. The pain was unbearable and she had missed a lot of school.

I explained that there was a good chance that removing her endometriosis would help the pain before her period, the pains during the month and the unexpected spots of blood. These symptoms were probably due to endometriosis. However, the severe pain on the first day of her period was a mixture of endometriosis and prostaglandin pain, so removing her endometriosis would not stop this. She would need other treatment for this pain. It was important that she understood that removing her endometriosis, although worthwhile, would not fix all her pain. Rosetta chose a laparoscopy to remove her endometriosis with a Mirena inserted at the same time.

Other causes of pain in teenagers

While 70 per cent of the teenagers with severe pelvic pain in the American study had endometriosis, 30 per cent did not. Not all pain is endometriosis, and pain can be a mixture of endometriosis and something else. Chapter 9 describes several other possible causes of pain. These apply to teenagers just as much as older women.

To make everything even worse, many teenagers are stressed or suffer depression. Young women, especially those with chronic pain, often have low self-esteem. They may be studying hard in their last year of school, or feeling anxious about their relationships, their family or their employment prospects. Others struggle with drug or alcohol dependence. The severe distress of sexual assault may also show as pelvic pain. *Just like endometriosis, stress and depression are often missed in teenagers.*

Exercise, maintaining a healthy weight, management of depression, a healthy diet and good self-esteem are so important, especially during the teenage years. While they may not treat the pain, they do prevent many of the other problems that women with pain suffer.

Why has it taken so long to recognise that teenagers get endometriosis?

For many years gynaecologists have been reluctant to do laparoscopies on teenagers. Teenagers were thought too young to have endometriosis. Unfortunately, this is not true. The youngest girl ever reported with endometriosis was ten and a half years old. No woman with periods is too young for endometriosis.

Even when a laparoscopy *is* done, endometriosis in teenagers is often missed. Clear, pink or red areas are much more common in teenagers than the easily seen brown or black lesions. Sometimes, the only abnormality found is an area with extra blood vessels or a pocket in the peritoneum (see Chapter 1, page 8). Endometriosis in teenagers is under-diagnosed.

I know I have endometriosis, but it wasn't removed

This is a very common situation, because many gynaecologists are not comfortable removing endometriosis at a laparoscopy. They have been trained to look for (diagnose) endometriosis, but not to remove it. This is particularly true if your endometriosis is severe.

At a first laparoscopy neither you, nor your gynaecologist, know what (if anything) will be found. If endometriosis *is* found, then your gynaecologist has to consider where your endometriosis is, the skills and resources available to them at the time, and the possible risks involved in removing the endometriosis. If removing endometriosis is not an operation they feel comfortable doing, or the staff, equipment or available time do not permit, then the endometriosis is usually left untreated.

This decision should be respected, because it is not in your interest to have surgery if the conditions are not right. The risk of complications is higher, and it can make later surgery more difficult.

Your laparoscopy has still been useful. You now have a diagnosis for your pain! This is the first step to effective treatment, but on its own will not help your pain. Which treatment you choose now depends on how troublesome your pain is, your own treatment preference and where the endometriosis was found. Unfortunately, it will also depend on the health services available to you.

Endometriosis removed as a two-stage procedure

Danielle is a 17-year-old woman from the country. Her periods were very painful and two days off school every month made it difficult for her to keep up with her schoolwork. A laparoscopy at her local hospital showed endometriosis. Her local gynaecologist recognised that her endometriosis should be removed, but knew that their local hospital was not equipped for such surgery. The extra time needed to recover from a more extensive laparoscopy would also mean even more time off school for Danielle.

Photographs from her laparoscopy were sent to our clinic for review. We agreed that Danielle needed her endometriosis removed and arranged a second laparoscopy in the city during her next school holidays. Danielle used the contraceptive pill continuously to avoid periods while waiting for her surgery.

What can I do about my endometriosis now?

Now you know that you have endometriosis, you can chose to have it removed, or choose to leave it and manage the pain in other ways. You may need to do both, because even removing endometriosis does not always mean that your pains go completely. Equally, endometriosis is not a life-threatening condition (even if it feels like it), so you could choose to do nothing.

Remember that any management choice should be just that. A choice. *Your choice.* Something you have decided on, together with your doctor, because *you* want help with *your* pain. Reasonable options to consider include:

- *A laparoscopy to completely remove the endometriosis, if that is possible.* This is a good option for women who know they have endometriosis. If the endometriosis is not completely removed (see Chapter 7, page 99), then you are more likely to find yourself in this situation again in the future.

- *Endometriosis medications.* There are special medications only offered to women who know that they have endometriosis. You were not eligible for them before your laparoscopy, but you are now. These medications are described more fully in Chapter 6. They work best on thin, active areas of endometriosis (the clear, pink or red lesions). They will not remove scar tissue, adhesions, nodules of endometriosis or chocolate cysts. A three to six month course of medication usually gives good pain relief for six to twelve months, but unfortunately pain often returns a few months after stopping the treatment. These medications do *not* improve fertility, and must not be taken while pregnant, so if becoming pregnant soon is your priority don't take them.

- *The contraceptive pill or a progestogen medication used continuously.* Neither medication will remove endometriosis, but they can cut down the number of periods you have each year. As fewer periods mean less period pain, they make it easier to live with your endometriosis. Both options work best for pain with periods or at ovulation. They are less helpful for pain at other times of the month. To have the least number of periods possible on the contraceptive pill, see Chapter 6, page 80.

- *A levonorgestrel intra-uterine device (Mirena) — see Chapter 6, page 77.* This is a newer option, but one that I believe will become more popular. It works best for pain that comes from the uterus, so might be useful as *part* of your plan.

- *Improved pain management.* Once again, this will not remove your endometriosis, but are you getting the most out of your pain medications? Is there something you haven't tried? Is there a better way of taking it? Your general practitioner can review your medications and offer ideas on what to take, and when. Common pain medications are discussed in Chapter 6, on page 65.

- *Complementary therapies.* This type of therapy is outside my area of expertise, but explained in a thoughtful way by Dr Margaret Taylor in Chapter 12. As knowledge of endometriosis varies widely between different herbal therapists, your general practitioner or endometriosis clinic may be able to recommend someone with whom they deal frequently. Endometriosis management requires co-operation, so pick someone who is comfortable working with your medical team.

- *Acupuncture.* I can only say that some of my patients have found it helpful. I look forward to the results of trials currently under way into acupuncture and period pain.

- *No treatment.* Maybe just knowing what has caused your pain is enough for you. It is important that you feel able to say no to treatment you don't want, whether it is medical, surgical or complementary.

In reality, you will probably need to look at more than one of these options to get the best result for your pain. You will also need to look at the stresses in your life. Period pain on a good day is period pain, but period pain on a bad day is unbearable. You need more good days!

The removal of endometriosis is not a procedure that all gynaecologists offer, so if you decide to have surgery, then now is the time to seek out the best surgical skills available to you. Endometriosis does not change quickly, so you have time. If you do plan to see another gynaecologist, they will need details from your previous laparoscopy. This information might include a copy of the operation sheet showing where your endometriosis is, photos taken at the laparoscopy (if available), or a copy of the letter sent to your general practitioner. If you have any of this information, keep it safely always. If you do not have this information, you can write to your surgeon or hospital requesting copies of the operation sheet. They will need your written, signed permission for this and it takes time, but this information is important. Your new doctor cannot plan your next laparoscopy well without it.

Whether or not a second laparoscopy is successful at improving your pain depends on how completely the endometriosis can be removed, and whether or not there are other causes for the pain.

> **Removing your endometriosis will only treat those symptoms that are due to the endometriosis. Symptoms from other causes will still be there after your surgery.**

Other ideas to improve your pain

- *Are there other health problems I can improve?* Most women with endometriosis have other problems too. These may be physical health problems or life stresses. Fixing any one problem will make it easier to live with the others. Is there something you *can* fix? For example, you may have periods that are heavy as well as painful. Any treatment that lightens your periods means fewer problems to deal with at period time.

- *Look after your mental health.* Any woman with pain benefits from time spent with a counsellor or psychologist. This is why I enjoy working with Jane Marsh so much. She is able to work through many issues that I, as a surgeon, feel ill equipped to handle. Frequently it is the women who were most reticent to see a counsellor who benefit the most.

- *Dietary changes.* Many women with endometriosis complain of bloating and bowel pain. If you already have pelvic pain from endometriosis, then the last thing you need is an irritable bowel to multiply the pain. Margaret Taylor writes on dietary management of pelvic pain in Chapter 12, on page 246 and bloating is discussed in Chapter 9 on page 169. A dietician may be able to check for food intolerances that could be causing your bowel symptoms.

- *Exercise.* Exercise makes us feel better because it releases natural pain killing chemicals called endorphins into our body *and* because it makes us stronger. Remember that the first couple of weeks of exercise just reminds the nerves and muscles how to work well together again. Improved health and strength comes with consistent exercise after this time. Is there exercise you *can* do, despite your pain?

My laparoscopy helped, but now the pain is back

To have had pain go and then come back is pretty depressing. The good news is that your pain improved before. It can improve again and this time, we hope, for longer.

To work out the best treatment for you, it is important to think about why the pain has come back. Generally, it will be for one of three reasons:

1   *Your endometriosis was not completely removed at your laparoscopy, and the remnants have become active again.* Removing endometriosis may be very difficult, so this is common. Cautery certainly reduces endometriosis, but may not remove it completely (see Chapter 7, page 99). Even the best endometriosis surgeons leave endometriosis behind sometimes. They may do this on purpose, particularly if these areas are near delicate structures that could be damaged.

2   *New areas of endometriosis have developed since your laparoscopy.* Endometriosis usually develops over a period of years during your teens and twenties. If you were only partly through this phase of your life at your last laparoscopy, then even after the best surgery new areas might develop. At the

first laparoscopy, some of the endometriosis you were destined to develop had not yet formed. If you have another laparoscopy now, new areas of endometriosis may be found in areas that looked normal last time. Unfortunately, only another laparoscopy will show whether there are new areas of endometriosis or not.

3 *Your pain is due to something else, not endometriosis.* Even if the pain feels similar to your old pain, it is always worth considering if it is a new pain (see Chapter 9).

The first two possibilities both mean that you might have endometriosis in your pelvis again, so the treatment options are the same as those in the earlier section on page 94.

The only difference is that if all your endometriosis *was* truly removed last time and you have now developed new areas of endometriosis, then a three to six months course of a GnRH analogue medication (see Chapter 6, page 67) may be worth trying. The new lesions have only been present a short time, so they are probably small, thin and few in number. These are the lesions most likely to respond to medications. If all goes well with the GnRH analogue, you may be able to avoid surgery. If not, then surgery remains an option.

Alternatively, another laparoscopy may be a good choice *if* the pain you have now is like your old pain, *and* your last laparoscopy really did help you, at least for a while. If your last laparoscopy did not help your pain at all, then consider other causes for your pain.

I think my endo has come back. Again!

Siobhan is a 25-year-old married woman with no children. Her first laparoscopy was done 4 years ago. Endometriosis was found and cauterised, but the pain she suffered for three in every four weeks only improved a little. Within a few months her pain was as bad as ever.

Two years ago she had her second laparoscopy. This time all her endometriosis was completely removed. Her pain was much improved for over a year. There was still pain on the first one or two days of her period, but this was pain from her uterus, rather than pain from endometriosis.

Two years later she returned. She had pain again and felt sure that more endometriosis must be present. A third laparoscopy showed no endometriosis at all. Her pain was now a mixture of bladder pain (see Chapter 9, page 188), neuropathic pain (see Chapter 9, page 177) and anxiety over her ability to have children rather than endometriosis. Siobhan felt relieved that her endometriosis had not returned, and moved on to manage the other causes of her pain.

If you do plan more surgery, it is a good idea to ask your gynaecologist what type of surgery would be done if endometriosis were found. It may be that an area of endometriosis was left behind at your last laparoscopy for a good reason. It may be close to important and easily damaged organs. Your next laparoscopy may be a much larger operation than your first. You need to know what would be involved and what risks there are.

How can I tell if my endometriosis was completely removed?

Complete removal of endometriosis from the pelvis means that at the end of the operation no endometriosis can be found. Endometriosis is removed in one of two ways.

The first technique is called *cautery* or *ablation*. It involves burning the top of any visible endometriosis lesions using electricity, laser or other instruments. It can remove small areas of endometriosis from the surface of the uterus or ovaries well, but is less successful in other areas. There are two reasons for this. First, as endometriosis usually lies close to important organs such as the ureter or bowel, gynaecologists tend to *under*-cauterise, rather than *over*-cauterise any lesions to avoid damaging these organs. This tends to take the top off a lesion but leave deeper areas behind, a bit like an iceberg where only part of the iceberg lies visible above the surface. Second, cautery only treats the spots of endometriosis that can be seen. Microscopic endometriosis in the areas between the endometriosis lesions are not cauterised because they look normal.

The second technique is called *excision* or *excisional surgery*. It can also be done with electricity, laser or other instruments, but rather than burning the top of the lesion, the whole lesion is cut out. With this comes the area of skin (peritoneum) around the endometriosis. Any microscopic areas are removed at the same time.

So, if your endometriosis was cauterised or ablated, it may or may not have been completely removed. If it was excised *and* your gynaecologist treated all the affected areas, then complete removal is more likely. *So unless your endometriosis is minor, or lies on the ovaries or uterus, complete removal really means excisional surgery rather than cautery.*

If you are not sure what type of surgery you have had, ask your doctor for details.

What other conditions could be causing my pain?

Other causes of pain in women who have had endometriosis are common. It is very difficult for most women to pick the cause of their pelvic pain because most sensations from the pelvis travel to the brain through similar pathways. This makes it difficult for your brain to decide which part of your pelvis the pain came from.

So, even if your current pain feels similar to the old pain, it may be due to a different condition. You may have two or more causes for your pain. Combinations such as endometriosis and bladder pain (interstitial cystitis), endometriosis and bowel pain, or endometriosis and neuropathic pain are very common. Chapter 9 includes details of how to pick what your pain might be.

The best treatment will depend on the cause of the pain.

Does endometriosis surgery work?

Yes, but not for all women, and not for all pain. An Australian study (Reference 16) asked 176 women to rate their pain as a score between 0 (no pain) and 10 (the worst pain imaginable) both before and after surgery for endometriosis. Period pain scores reduced from an average of 9 before surgery to 3 after surgery. It did not take away all their period pain, but they were certainly better. In women with daily pelvic pain, the pain score fell from 8 to 3, and for women with pain opening their bowels from 7 to 2. The best result was a fall in pain score from 7 to 0 in women with painful intercourse. *These women had expert excisional surgery.* Over a two to five year period, one in three women had further surgery looking for endometriosis, but new endometriosis was only found in two-thirds of these women. The other one-third had pain like endometriosis, but no endometriosis was found.

My endometriosis was removed, but I still have pain

Few things are as disappointing or demoralising as continued pain after an operation you thought would solve your problems. *Why has it happened? Why aren't I better?* In most cases it is a mixture of the complicated nature of pelvic pain, the limitations of surgery and unrealistic expectations (yours or your doctor's) of what surgery can achieve.

This is where the modern management of pelvic pain still needs improvement. As endometriosis surgeons, we have believed that if we could just develop our surgical skills enough, that we could cure our patients' pelvic pain. Sometimes we can, but sometimes we can't. As a surgeon, I believe it is important that I give women a realistic expectation of what can be achieved with surgery. Doctors *want* to help women in pain. They also want to believe that they *can* help women in pain. Women *want* to believe that their pain can be cured. It is easy for unrealistic expectations to develop on both sides. Sometimes the pain *is* gone after surgery, but often an operation is one (important) part of a complete treatment plan. Getting the best results usually means a mix of treatments as well as some lifestyle changes.

Surgery for any condition usually involves *repairing* the body, or *removing* an organ. Even the best repair is just that, *a repair*. Surgery to remove endometriosis can repair the pelvis and, we hope, treat those pains that are due to endometriosis, but it cannot make a new pelvis, nor treat pain from other causes. Even though you had endometriosis this does not mean that this was the only cause for your pain. Not all endometriosis is painful and most women have more than one cause for their pain. This is where it is important to keep in mind the other causes of pelvic pain described in Chapter 9.

What else could the pain be?

Think about your pain. You may notice that your pain is different now. It may come at different times of the month or feel different in some way. Some symptoms may have improved, while others have not. Before your surgery, you may have had two causes of pain, both sending pain impulses to your brain through the same nerve pathways. After your surgery, one cause was removed, but the other cause is still there and is still sending pain signals through the same pathways. Not surprisingly, your brain may feel as though little has changed.

How the brain feels pain and the pain pathways are explained further in Chapter 9, on page 146.

In general, painful periods with good health for the rest of the month might be prostaglandin pain (page 155), adenomyosis (page 151), clot colic or pelvic congestion syndrome (page 198).

Pain present on most days over a long period of time is called *chronic pain*. Chronic pain *and* bladder symptoms might mean interstitial cystitis. Chronic pain that is worse with certain movements or a change in activity may be muscular or joint pain. Pain with a 'burning' or 'sharp' quality may be neuropathic pain and pain with diarrhoea, constipation or bloating may be bowel pain. Adenomyosis can cause either daily pain or period pain.

As well as describing all of these conditions more fully, Chapter 9 also suggests people who can help you with these pains.

Remember that these suggestions presume that there is now no endometriosis left in your pelvis. If your endometriosis was not completely removed, then managing your pain becomes more complicated. To move forward, you need to know what is left and what type of surgery was done. If some endometriosis has been left behind, this does not mean that you have been managed badly by your gynaecologist. It may well have been the best decision at the time considering the skills available and the risks involved.

My doctor said my endometriosis is 'mild', but it still hurts (a lot!)

Catarina is a 38-year-old married woman who would like to have a baby. She has always had painful periods and after two years of trying to get pregnant had a laparoscopy with her gynaecologist. The operation report described only a few spots of endometriosis, but scarring involving both uterosacral ligaments and several adhesions. The brown lesions had been cauterised and some of the adhesions divided, but her pain continued. To me, this usually means that there is more endometriosis present than first realised.

Catarina had no other cause for adhesions apart from endometriosis and yet the amount of endometriosis described did not sound enough to cause so many adhesions. At her second laparoscopy there were a few spots of brown endometriosis, several adhesions around both ovaries, and thick white scarring of both uterosacral ligaments. All the scar tissue, the endometriosis and the adhesions were cut out completely and all showed endometriosis when checked by a pathologist. Whether or not she becomes pregnant will depend on many things (see Chapter 8, page 119), but we hope she will at least have less pain.

How to avoid feelings of abandonment

After all the time spent with your doctors during the diagnosis and treatment of your endometriosis, it is easy to feel abandoned once treatment finishes. Couples who use IVF to become pregnant have similar problems. There is a flurry of activity, but once they become pregnant they are on their own. There is little contact with those people who were once a regular part of their life.

An endometriosis specialist may not offer general gynaecological reviews, and may not feel able to help manage other causes of pain once your endometriosis has been treated. Your general practitioner remains the key to coordinating your care. This is one reason why it is so important to have a general practitioner with whom you have a long-term professional relationship. Some ways to avoid feeling abandoned include:

- An after-treatment appointment with your counsellor, if one was involved with your care. Just because the pain is better, relationships do not always improve, nor jobs become more satisfying.

- A regular monthly visit to your general practitioner until you are truly well. Questions and concerns can be stored up over this time and the stress of 'Do I, or don't I need to see the doctor' is avoided.
- Plan a review visit with your endometriosis surgeon 6 months after your surgery. It will take this long to work out which symptoms are better and which are not, especially if you are spacing periods out with the contraceptive pill. Keep a list of questions ready to ask at your visit. If no endometriosis was found, or your surgeon has nothing more to offer, ask whom you should see for further advice.

Endometriosis is in our family

Some women know all about endometriosis. Their mother, sister, or aunt has suffered and not surprisingly they are worried. Endometriosis *is* more common in families, but just because you have a relative with endometriosis, it does not mean that you will get it too. Even if you do, there is more to offer now.

No-one fully understands how endometriosis is inherited, but some things are becoming clearer.

It seems likely that whether or not a woman inherits a tendency to endometriosis probably involves many different genes. Some things about us (like our eye colour) probably involve only one pair of genes: one gene from each parent. If one of these genes is for brown eyes, then you *will* have brown eyes. There are few other factors involved.

Endometriosis is different. There are probably many genes involved. None of these genes on its own decides whether or not you will get endometriosis, but the more of these 'endometriosis risk' genes you have, the more likely it is that you will. Each gene increases the risk a little. This inheritance is similar to the way asthma or diabetes is inherited in families.

Women with severe endometriosis probably have many 'endometriosis risk' genes. Because they have so many, there is a good chance that their relatives will share at least some of these genes too. This may explain why the chance of having endometriosis is higher if you have a relative with severe endometriosis, than if you have a relative with mild endometriosis. Women with mild endometriosis may only have a few 'endometriosis risk' genes.

Genetics is an exciting area of medicine that is changing rapidly. Within the next few years, it may be able to explain which genes are involved and better predict which women are at highest risk of developing endometriosis.

Whatever our genes, other environmental factors are important too. Some women with endometriosis have no relatives with endometriosis, and other women with a strong family history of endometriosis never have problems.

What is the risk of endometriosis in twins?

An Australian study of twins (see Reference 16) showed that where one *identical twin* had endometriosis, the other twin had endometriosis too 30 per cent of the time. Identical twins share the same genes because they came from the same egg. These results show that our genes play a major part in whether or not we develop endometriosis, but that other factors are important too. If our genes were the only factor, then if one twin had endometriosis, the other twin should have it too in 100 per cent of cases, not just 30 per cent.

Just what these other factors are is not well understood.

If a *non-identical* twin has endometriosis, then the other twin is affected only 10 per cent of the time. This is because non-identical twins only share some genes. Their risk of endometriosis is similar to the risk other children in their family have.

Sisters with endometriosis

Alex was 14 when she came with her mother requesting a laparoscopy. Fourteen is young to have endometriosis, but her pain was severe. Alex herself felt sure of the diagnosis. Her much older sister Valerie suffered severe period pain from the age of 15, but was only diagnosed with endometriosis at 21 when she finally had her first laparoscopy. Before then she was considered 'too young for endometriosis'. Endometriosis has been a continuing problem for Valerie. Alex recognised the symptoms, and wanted to act quickly.

At laparoscopy Alex's endometriosis was widespread and completely removed. She became my youngest patient with endometriosis. Time will tell whether excising her endometriosis completely and promptly, will lessen the major problems her sister has had.

Nothing seems to work for me

Chronic pain despite everything is miserable. This is where endometriosis gets really hard. There is a small group of women for whom no treatment has provided lasting benefit. Over many years their episodes of acute period pain have become daily, chronic pain. Fewer women need suffer this now, but some still do.

If you have severe chronic pain, there is really no choice but to continue looking for ways to improve or cope with the pain. The option of 'just ignoring it' is unrealistic unless your pain is minor. However, there may come a time when you have run out of ideas.

If this is your story, I do not pretend to have all the answers, but the following section has some ideas for a fresh start.

First of all, has all your endometriosis *truly* been completely removed? If you don't know, ask your gynaecologist.

Ideas if you still have endometriosis present

- *Obtain as many details of your previous surgery and endometriosis treatments as you can and seek out the best endometriosis surgeon available to you.* Any surgery now is likely to be difficult.

- *If further surgery is not a realistic option, then consider one of the newer anti-endometriosis medications discussed in Chapter 6.* Over time, more information on which of these are effective and safe will become available. There are very few women in whom surgery to remove endometriosis is truly not an option, but the surgery required may be major and does have the risk of significant complications.

- *Review again the options on pages 93–97 or Chapter 9.*

Ideas if all your endometriosis is gone

- *What actually is causing the pain?* Your pain may have started as endometriosis pain but changed over the years into pain from something else. You are no longer an 'endometriosis patient'. You are a woman with chronic pain. Read all the types of pain in Chapter 9, and see which fit with your pain.

- *Try pregabalin or amitriptyline.* (See Chapter 6, pages 72 and 74). These medications are often effective in women with pain on most days. They are well worth trying. If one does not help you, try the other one.

- *Try a Mirena IUD.* (See Chapter 6, page 77). This is especially useful if your pain is severe on the first 1 or 2 days of your period.

- *Could a pain management specialist or pain clinic help?* Pain management is a specialty in itself. A pain specialist manages chronic pain from many causes, of which endometriosis is just one. He or she has knowledge and medications that are outside your gynaecologist's experience. You will need to take details of your previous surgery with you, particularly those describing your most recent laparoscopy.

- *Are there emotional issues holding back your progress?* No operation or tablet will heal the hurt of infertility, low self-esteem or sexual assault. Tackle the issues complicating your pain. Review your general health, and life stresses. A psychologist, endometriosis counsellor or occupational therapist can help.

- *Is it time to consider a major operation?* Some women only improve after surgery to remove the uterus, any scar tissue, any remaining endometriosis, and sometimes both ovaries. This is a big decision and not reasonable for young women, women who would like to have children, or women who need their uterus to feel good about their body. If you have completed your family, and particularly if you also have heavy periods, an operation such as this may be a good choice. *Remember that a hysterectomy alone, without removal of any remaining endometriosis is not enough.* Before considering an operation such as this you need to feel confident that any abnormal areas in the pelvis will be removed. You must also feel sure that your pain *does* actually have a gynaecological cause. To have a major operation and find that the pain is still present would be disappointing to say the least!

> **A complete cure for chronic pain may not be possible, but worthwhile improvement in the pain almost always is.**

You may find that many of your life goals can still be achieved, even if some of your pain remains. Some occupational therapists specialise in helping people live with chronic pain. They can work with you on what you *can* achieve; to help you maintain or resume the parts of your life that have always been important to you.

It is not surprising that many women with chronic pain become focused on their pain. Many lose sight of the 'non-pain goals' in their life. Before the pain, they had many interests and pleasures. Now there is only the quest for a cure. Maintaining one's personality and appreciation of life is a challenge when confronted with daily pain. Some women succeed. They are inspiring and unsung heroes.

Anger and disappointment after years of pain

Annie is a 45-year-old woman who has always had painful periods. No treatment for her endometriosis had helped. She married at 35, and tried to become pregnant without success. After three failed cycles of fertility treatment, and at 40 years of age, she and her husband decided to accept that a pregnancy was unlikely and stopped trying. Despite knowing that logically she should move on in her life, the bitter disappointment of living without children had never left her. Her experience of medical care had been disappointing, and left her angry. It had delivered her neither pain relief nor children. When we first met, she was angry and suffered daily pain, much worse with periods.

After a discussion of the treatments she had had in the past, Annie felt better. She now understood that although inadequate for her needs, she had at least been offered the best that was available at the time. We discussed what pain management options she had left. These included:

- *A laparoscopy to look for and remove any remaining endometriosis.* At 45 years of age and after previous surgery there was probably no endometriosis left. Her current pain was much more likely to be a combination of adenomyosis, adhesions or neuropathic pain. A laparoscopy alone would only remove any remaining endometriosis, and divide any adhesions. It was unlikely to manage all her pain.

- *A laparoscopic hysterectomy with removal of any remaining endometriosis, any scar tissue, possibly her ovaries, and then the option of HRT if she chose to use it.* Medically, this was the option most likely to help her pain. However, emotionally this would mean confronting her childless state, and putting aside any chance of pregnancy, no matter how small. Annie was a long way from this decision.
- *Medications to improve pain* such as amitriptyline, period pain medications taken regularly, a continuous oral contraceptive pill or a progestogen medication.
- *Referral to a pain management specialist.*

It is important to me as a gynaecologist that women want their surgery. *If they don't want it, I don't want to do it.* Annie was not ready for any of these options. She needed time to think. After speaking with Jane Marsh, Annie decided to work through her emotional needs with a psychologist before considering any surgery. Annie is welcome to return if she chooses to.

Removal of the uterus, ovaries, endometriosis and scar tissue for chronic pelvic pain

Antonia is a 35-year-old woman with a long history of severe endometriosis managed very competently elsewhere. She and her husband, Bill, had healthy six-year-old triplets, conceived using IVF, and no plan for more children. While on a family holiday, Antonia's pain became worse. She always had some pain, but this pain was so severe they were unable to continue their trip. All the surgery possible through a laparoscope had been done. Antonia had thick scar tissue between her bowel, uterus, and ovaries. Despite her young age she felt ready for major surgery. Antonia decided to have a hysterectomy with removal of all her scar tissue, a segment of bowel affected by endometriosis and both ovaries. It was a difficult operation done with the help of a bowel surgeon. All the scar tissue was removed, but the surgery required a large cut on her abdomen. After the operation, Antonia recovered well and left hospital 8 days later. Both oestrogen and testosterone replacement medication were started as she was only 35 years old, and her ovaries had been removed. Oestrogen replacement avoids hot flushes and other menopausal symptoms. Testosterone replacement avoids the tiredness and low libido common in young women whose ovaries have been removed.

Three weeks after surgery, Antonia developed crampy abdominal pains, vomiting and a swollen abdomen. She was admitted to hospital with a blockage in the bowel (called a 'bowel obstruction'). This settled after a few days of fasting and fluid through a drip. A temporary bowel blockage like this sometimes occurs after surgery near the bowel but usually settles without surgery. We hope it will not recur. Antonia continued on her family trip 6 weeks later with much less pain than before and the promise of no more periods.

Chapter 8

Frequently asked questions

What causes endometriosis?

N O-ONE KNOWS what causes endometriosis, but several possibilities have been suggested.

Most doctors, if asked, will put forward *'Sampson's theory'* which dates from 1921. Sampson noticed that women who had operations during their period often had period (menstrual) blood in their pelvis at the time of their operation. This blood flowed through the fallopian tubes into the pelvis, rather than out through the vagina. This process is called *'retrograde menstruation'* and is normal for most women.

Sampson's explanation was that live fragments of endometrium (lining of the uterus) mixed with the period blood, settled around the pelvic organs, implanted on the surface of these organs and grew into endometriosis. Several factors fitted this theory. It was noted that endometriosis does not occur in girls before menstruation begins, and that endometriosis is more common in those rare women with a blockage in their cervix that prevents their menstrual blood flowing into the vagina normally.

However, there are many factors that do *not* fit with Sampson's theory:

- An endometriosis lesion is *not* the same as endometrium (the lining of the uterus). It is only similar to it in some ways.
- Endometriosis may be found in places outside the pelvis, such as the lung. It is found in rare cases in men who have used oesatrogen medications to treat cancer of the prostate. Endometriosis in these areas cannot be due to retrograde menstruation.
- Genetic tests on areas of endometriosis show that they have a different origin from endometrial tissue from the same woman. If the endometriosis came from cells spread from the uterus, they should be genetically the same.
- Endometriosis usually develops during a woman's teens or twenties, after only a few years of periods. New endometriosis developing after this is less common. If Sampson's theory were true, then as time goes by and more periods occur the likelihood of new endometriosis should continue to increase.

Sampson lived in 1921, before much of the modern medical knowledge we now take for granted.

So, what other possible causes are there?

Even before the genetics of endometriosis were better understood, came an alternative theory. The *Metaplasia theory* suggests that some cells in the peritoneum lining the pelvis are predestined to change (metaplase) into endometriosis once conditions are right.

Which factors bring about the right conditions? Once again, no-one knows, but one factor appears to be the rise in oesatrogen level that occurs with puberty. There are probably others that affect in whom and when endometriosis lesions form, but as yet they are poorly understood.

One of these factors probably involves the immune system, but exactly how this happens remains unclear. Women with endometriosis are more likely to develop illnesses to do with the immune system, but many don't. Research has found other immune differences between women with and without endometriosis too, but so far it has not been easy to put all the known facts together. Research into this area continues.

Another factor may be our environment. Some toxins, such as dioxin (found in air pollution) have been linked to endometriosis.

So which one is the real cause?

It is possible that all these theories have some truth in them.

Endometriosis may be a collection of disorders, each with a different mix of causes. There may be one type of endometriosis due to retrograde menstruation and another due to metaplasia, both influenced by changes in the immune system, the environment and our hormones. There is a lot more to be learned about what causes endometriosis and what causes pelvic pain where no endometriosis is found.

One thing is certain. You cannot 'catch' endometriosis. It is not contagious like an infection, and cannot be passed from one person to another.

What about endometriosis in the rectovaginal septum?

Doctors disagree on how rectovaginal endometriosis forms (see Figure 5.1, page 40). No period blood reaches here, so it is not due to retrograde menstruation (Sampson's theory). Some doctors believe that it is due to metaplasia: that it forms from cells that have been there since birth and then turned into endometriosis when the time was right. Others believe that endometriosis here is really a type of adenomyosis (see Chapter 9, page 151), and thus a different disease altogether.

Can endometriosis be prevented?

Whether or not you believe that endometriosis can be prevented, depends on what you believe causes endometriosis in the first place (see our earlier discussion in this chapter).

If you believe that endometriosis is caused by retrograde menstruation then any treatment that cuts down the number of periods or the amount of blood passing into the pelvis should decrease the chance of endometriosis. Less blood means less opportunity for endometrial cells from inside the uterus to settle in the pelvis.

However, if endometriosis is caused by metaplasia, then the number of periods and amount of blood passed into the pelvis may not matter. Those areas of peritoneum that are destined to become endometriosis in some women will do so, once a suitable environment is present for endometriosis to grow. The only prevention possible is a change in the environmental or immune factors that stimulate the growth of endometriosis. Some of these factors might be changes in hormone levels or avoiding exposure to toxins in our environment. Much more needs to be known about what actually does promote its growth.

The metaplasia theory includes both good and not-so-good news. The not-so-good news is that prevention of endometriosis may not be possible (for now, at least). Endometriosis that is destined to develop will do so if the conditions for its growth are right. The good news is that once an affected area of peritoneum affected by endometriosis has been excised, the peritoneum that grows over the area will be healthy new peritoneum that is unlikely to develop new endometriosis. This is what I see in my patients. In places where endometriosis has been completely excised (not just cauterised) it rarely recurs. Any new endometriosis is usually found in areas of peritoneum that were not removed before, because they looked normal.

Factors encouraging the growth of endometriosis in some women, but not others, are poorly understood. Women with habits that lower oestrogen levels, such as exercise, have a lower chance of developing endometriosis (see Reference 10). Regular exercise during the teenage years has other health benefits as well, and is highly recommended.

The Pill may also help. It prevents the high levels of oestrogen present during ovulation. So, even though the Pill is an oestrogen medication, women who take it often have a lower overall oestrogen level than women who do not. An Australian study concluded that women who use the Pill for more than five years have a 30 per cent less chance of developing endometriosis than those not taking the Pill (see Reference 10).

Will my endometriosis come back?

It might, but if it is completely removed, there is a good chance that it will not return.

Many women have been told that 'You can't cure endometriosis — it always comes back'. I do not believe this statement, but I do accept that, even after the best surgery, new areas may form. Understandably, women who have suffered severe pain in the past, then found relief from the pain may worry that their pain will return.

An Australian study (see Reference 15) followed the progress of 250 women for between two and five years after laparoscopic excision of their endometriosis. Of these, 36 per cent had another operation over this time. Another operation was especially likely if their endometriosis was severe at their first laparoscopy. However, only two-thirds of the women who did have more surgery actually had endometriosis found at their next operation. This means that about *one in four* women had new areas of endometriosis develop over this time.

Personally, I believe that the likelihood that new areas of endometriosis will develop after it has been removed is higher in younger women.

I believe that most endometriosis develops during a woman's teens and twenties. If her endometriosis is removed *after* all the endometriosis she was destined to make has formed, then it is less likely that new areas will grow. She may develop pain from a different cause (see Chapter 9), but new areas of endometriosis itself are uncommon.

However, if her laparoscopy was done *before* all her endometriosis had formed, then the chance of finding new areas at a second laparoscopy is higher. Her first operation could only remove the endometriosis that was visible at the time. When new endometriosis forms, it is usually found in the areas that looked normal last time, rather than in the areas treated at her first operation.

> **So, the younger you are when your endometriosis is first diagnosed and removed, the higher the chance that new areas of endometriosis will develop in the future. The older you are when your endometriosis is removed, the lower the chance that *new* areas of endometriosis will form.**

All of this presumes that the endometriosis has been removed completely. Endometriosis that has been cauterised or laser ablated (rather than laser excised) may improve for a short time, but is more likely to recur. Some women have many laparoscopies, each with cautery, a short improvement and then a recurrence of their pain. This is why many people believe that endometriosis always comes back. Cautery remains a useful treatment for lesions on the surface of the ovaries or uterus, or very thin lesions elsewhere.

When a woman who has had endometriosis in the past gets pain, it is often presumed to be due to endometriosis. This may or may not be true. The pelvis feels many pains in a similar way, so it is easy to be confused about what is actually causing the pain, especially when it is a mixture of different pains. A woman such as this is described in Chapter 9, on page 187, and information about other causes of pain are also described in Chapter 9.

Recurrence of endometriosis in a young woman

Simone came to see me first when she was 22. Her periods were irregular and painful. A laparoscopy showed endometriosis, which was completely removed, and her pain improved. Taking the contraceptive pill made her periods regular and avoided the prostaglandin pain that is usual in most women without children.

Three years later, Simone returned for review. Her pain was coming back despite the contraceptive pill. A laparoscopy showed new areas of endometriosis but only in areas that were normal the first time. The areas removed previously looked healthy. The new endometriosis was once again removed completely and her pain became manageable again. It is hoped that she has now produced all the endometriosis she is destined to develop, and there will be no further recurrence.

Will I be able to have children?

Many women with endometriosis fall pregnant easily. However, others find it difficult to become pregnant. Why?

Becoming pregnant is a complex process. Endometriosis is one factor not in your favour when trying to become pregnant. However, there are so many other factors involved that, if everything else is normal, you may never have a problem becoming pregnant. These other factors include the quality of the man's sperm, the woman's age, whether or not she ovulates each month, and whether or not her fallopian tubes are open.

Most couples who find it difficult to become pregnant have either severe endometriosis present, or other problems apart from the endometriosis.

Possible problems might include a low sperm count, or irregular periods with infrequent ovulation. When two or more 'minor' problems add together, becoming pregnant becomes much harder to achieve. For example, a common situation is a woman with mild endometriosis, and a man with a slightly lower than normal sperm count. Neither problem is severe on its own, but together the chance of becoming pregnant becomes less.

However, even couples with a mixture of fertility problems do become pregnant sometimes. I almost never say that pregnancy is impossible, just unlikely without help.

Once a woman does become pregnant, endometriosis will not hurt her baby. All pregnancies have a chance that the baby may not develop normally, but endometriosis does not increase this chance.

How does endometriosis affect fertility?

This depends on how severe the endometriosis is.

For many years, doctors have disagreed whether mild endometriosis with no scarring of the pelvis has any effect on fertility at all. Although some doctors still believe that mild endometriosis has no effect, most believe that it does affect fertility, but are unsure why. Several possibilities have been suggested. These include a changed environment for the egg or sperm, an effect on ovulation, a toxic effect on the newly formed embryo, or an effect on the hormones made by the ovary.

When there is severe endometriosis present, it is easy to understand how fertility could be affected. It can cause scarring that can block the fallopian tubes, prevent normal ovulation, or prevent the fallopian tubes picking up the egg once it is released. It can also make intercourse too painful to consider. Luckily, most women with endometriosis do not have scarring like this.

Can treatments for endometriosis improve my fertility?

Most doctors believe that an operation to remove any endometriosis, whether it is mild or severe, does improve fertility. The chance of becoming pregnant increases by about 40 per cent after surgical removal of endometriosis, and the first six months after the operation seem to be a particularly fertile time.

So, if your endometriosis is removed, you may be able to avoid the need for more complicated fertility treatments such as IVF. Even if IVF is still required, it is more likely to be successful if your endometriosis is removed first.

Medical therapies such as GnRH analogues, progestogens or danazol (see Chapter 6) *do not* improve fertility. They also take up valuable time, because pregnancy must be avoided during treatment.

What is JVF?

In-vitro fertilisation (IVF) means fertilisation of the egg by sperm in a laboratory, rather than in the body. Eggs are collected from the woman, and a semen sample is collected from the man. The eggs and sperm are mixed together in a dish, allowing the sperm to fertilise the eggs. Between one and three fertilised eggs are then inserted into the woman's uterus.

Becoming pregnant normally is a complex process. Sperm must be deposited in the vagina, penetrate the mucus in the cervix, travel up through the fallopian tubes, and penetrate the outer covering of an egg. There must be an egg ready for the sperm to fertilise. The fertilised egg must then travel back down the fallopian tube to the uterus and implant there.

IVF can help if there are problems with any of these steps.

Low sperm count and endometriosis

Angela is 32 years old. She and her husband Tom began investigation of their fertility after a year of trying to conceive was unsuccessful. Tom was found to have a very low sperm count. Angela ovulated regularly. No laparoscopy was done as Angela had only mild period pain, and it was thought that Tom's low sperm count was their only problem. However, after three unsuccessful cycles of IVF, Angela's fertility doctor wondered if there might be some endometriosis present and referred her to me for a laparoscopy. Although Angela had very little pain, a laparoscopy showed several areas of endometriosis that were then completely removed. Her fallopian tubes were normal and open. Angela and Tom will still need IVF due to his low sperm count. However, their chance of a successful pregnancy with each IVF cycle is increased now that her endometriosis has been removed.

When to ask for investigation of infertility

When you want to become pregnant, every month that goes by feels like one month too many. You may have friends who all seem to get pregnant easily, or all seem to be having babies. It is very stressful waiting to see if you will become pregnant, and worrying that there may be a problem.

Even if all your friends do seem to become pregnant easily, many couples don't. The chance of becoming pregnant after one month of intercourse without contraception is actually only 20 per cent. This means that only one in five couples will become pregnant after one month without contraception. After 12 months of trying, four in five couples will have become pregnant. That means that after a year, one in five couples will be disappointed.

If you have not become pregnant after 12 months of trying to do so, you may wish to discuss your fertility with your doctor. Although some couples would become pregnant without help if they waited another year, 12 months is considered a good time to start any investigations.

However, if you or your partner already know of a reason why becoming pregnant might be difficult, you may wish to talk to your general practitioner or gynaecologist earlier. Irregular periods, a known low sperm count, or where the woman is over 35 years of age are good examples of this.

When is the best time of the month to get pregnant?

Pregnancy is most likely if you have sex at ovulation. This is the time when the ovary releases an egg and you notice a large amount of clear, stretchy, jelly-like mucus. Intercourse every couple of days around ovulation time is enough because your partner needs to replenish his semen count between times.

How can I tell if I am ovulating?

A month where an egg is released from the ovary is called an *ovulatory cycle*. Some women know they are having ovulatory cycles. They have all the telltale signs. Others are less sure, or don't know what to look for.

Think about your periods. Ovulatory cycles are usually regular. This means that the number of days between the first day of one period and the first day of the next period is about the same each month. Ovulatory cycles are usually between 21 and 35 days long.

> **If you have *regular* periods, the day when ovulation should occur can be worked out by the formula:**
>
> Day of ovulation = Cycle length – 14
>
> If your period comes every 28 days, then you probably ovulate on day 14 (28 – 14 = 14).
>
> If your period comes every 35 days, then you probably ovulate on day 21 (35 – 14 = 21).

Check your vaginal mucus. Ovulatory cycles have clear, plentiful and stretchy vaginal mucus for two or three days leading up to ovulation. This change is due to rising oestrogen levels. After ovulation the mucus becomes less, whiter, and thicker.

Measure your temperature every morning. A temperature chart filled in each morning shows a 0.2–0.5 degree increase in body temperature after ovulation. Although this is an effective way to tell if ovulation has taken place, I don't recommend temperature charts because this daily reminder of infertility is emotionally stressful and time consuming. A progesterone blood test taken seven days before a period is more reliable and simpler.

Have your progesterone level checked. Progesterone is a hormone made by the ovary in the second half of a normal ovulatory cycle, *if* an egg has been released from the ovary that month. In cycles where no egg is released, there is no progesterone hormone made by the ovary. A blood test for progesterone, taken seven days before a period starts, will tell if ovulation has occurred that month or not. If ovulation did occur, the progesterone level will be high. If ovulation did not occur, the progesterone level will be low. The blood test result only applies to the month in which it is taken. It does not tell whether you will ovulate next month or not.

I have irregular periods. Can I become pregnant?

Some women don't ovulate as regularly as others. They still ovulate but it doesn't happen on the same day each month. This makes predicting ovulation a bit trickier, but pregnancy is certainly possible. There may be some months where no egg is released at all. These are called *anovulatory cycles*. All women have anovulatory cycles sometimes, but some women have them more often than others. Remember that even women with very few periods ovulate sometimes, so pregnancy is not impossible, even if there have been no periods for some time.

Professor Robert Jansen's book *Getting Pregnant* has detailed information on all aspects of fertility (see Reference 17).

I have endometriosis and don't want to become pregnant. Do I need contraception?

Yes, definitely. If you do *not* want to become pregnant you must use reliable contraception. Never presume that your endometriosis will prevent a pregnancy, even in a very scarred pelvis.

If less reliable methods of contraception have worked well for you in the past, they may not be as reliable once your endometriosis has been removed. Your fertility may increase and you may need to review your contraception.

An unplanned pregnancy after removal of endometriosis

Cassandra is a 30-year-old single farmer. Her periods were regular, and very painful. Although very keen to avoid a pregnancy, she and her partner used condoms, without spermicide, for contraception. Cassandra had used this contraception successfully for years, and was unwilling to consider a more reliable method. A laparoscopy to investigate her period pain found moderate endometriosis, which was completely removed and her pain improved.

Six months later, Cassandra came back for review. She was two months into an unplanned pregnancy, and one month after a

split with her boyfriend. Fertility improves after removal of
endometriosis even in those who don't want it. After a lot of
thought, Cassandra continued with the pregnancy alone.

If you are young, and not even thinking of children for now,
you should presume that you could get pregnant easily. If you do
have problems one day, it is possible that you may need fertility
assistance. However, this is true for many couples, not just those
with endometriosis. All women are advised to have babies earlier
rather than later if they are socially able to do so, because fertility
does decrease with age. Leaving pregnancies until you are in your
late thirties will work for some women, but will leave others
disappointed.

Will I need a hysterectomy?

Most women with endometriosis do *not* need a hysterectomy.

A hysterectomy is an operation to remove the uterus. It is not a
treatment for endometriosis because these lesions usually lie
outside the uterus. Removing the uterus but leaving endometriosis
behind is unlikely to make your endometriosis go away, and may
not help your pain.

However, there are other causes of pelvic pain that a hysterectomy *does* treat well. These causes include adenomyosis (see
Chapter 9, page 151), prostaglandins (see Chapter 9, page 155),
and pelvic congestion (see Chapter 9, page 198). They all cause
pain that feels similar to the pain of endometriosis, but is in fact
coming from the uterus. Many women have both endometriosis
and pain from their uterus. Removing the endometriosis is still the
best treatment for endometriosis, but adding a hysterectomy is one
way of treating pain from the uterus as well.

A hysterectomy becomes even more reasonable in women

who have no plan for future pregnancy, but have other conditions such as heavy periods or troublesome fibroids (see page 128). There are also a few women with very severe endometriosis in whom surgery is easier when the uterus is removed at the same time as their endometriosis.

Even so, you should never feel that you have to have a hysterectomy. With modern surgical techniques, it is almost always possible to remove the endometriosis without removing the uterus. In general, a hysterectomy in women under the age of 35 is rarely necessary. Women who wish to conserve their uterus, for whatever reason, should be able to do so. Their pain management may be more difficult in some cases, but neither adenomyosis, nor prostaglandin pain, are life-threatening conditions. Unless you have a cancer you never have to have a hysterectomy. Even heavy bleeding with periods can usually be managed in other ways. A hysterectomy should always be a choice, made by you, after consideration of the options available.

Women who have never had serious pelvic problems find it hard to believe that a woman would ever want to lose her uterus. Many women who have suffered for years can't wait to do so. We are all different, and our views on hysterectomy depend on our age, fertility, cultural background, and life experience.

Some women choose a hysterectomy, even if this is not absolutely necessary. Their lives have been dictated by pain and bleeding. Social activities depend on the time of the month. Holidays are difficult or impossible. They wish to move on in their lives, and leave periods behind. This is entirely reasonable. Very few women in this situation regret their decision. The vast majority of such women comment afterwards: 'I should have done it years ago.' Hysterectomy remains a popular operation for women with period pain, heavy periods and completed families.

> **Remember that a hysterectomy alone does not remove endometriosis. If the uterus is removed, but the endometriosis is left behind, your pain may continue.**

What is the difference between a hysterectomy and a 'full' hysterectomy?

Actually there is no difference. A hysterectomy is an operation to remove the uterus. The ovaries are conserved.

The word 'full' is often used by non-medical people to describe an operation where both the uterus *and* the ovaries are removed. This is not correct. A full hysterectomy (from a medical viewpoint) means a hysterectomy where both the cervix (lower part of the uterus) and the body (upper part of the uterus) are removed. This is distinct from a 'partial' or 'subtotal' hysterectomy where the body of the uterus is removed, but the cervix is left behind.

If the ovaries are removed, the operation is called a 'bilateral oophorectomy'. Bilateral means both sides. If the fallopian tubes are removed at the same time, it is called a **bilateral salpingo-oophorectomy**. So, an operation where the uterus, both fallopian tubes and both ovaries are removed is described as a 'hysterectomy with bilateral salpingo-oophorectomy'. If you are having a hysterectomy, you should be clear what will be removed and what will be kept.

What are fibroids?

Fibroids are tumours that grow in the muscle wall of the uterus. Only about 1 in 1000 fibroids are cancerous, so almost all are benign (not cancerous). The medical name for a fibroid is *leiomyoma*, and they are sometimes called *myomas*. Fibroids are common. Up to 30 per cent of women will have fibroids by the time they are 40, but many of these are small and not significant.

Fibroids vary a great deal in size. They range from less than 1 cm to several cm across. Fibroids only need removal if they cause symptoms such as heavy periods, or pressure on nearby organs like the bladder or bowel.

The site of the fibroid is very important. A woman with a small fibroid on the inside of her uterus may have very heavy periods, despite its small size. A woman with a large fibroid on the outside of the uterus may have normal periods, but notice pressure on her bladder or bowel.

Hysterectomy after years of pain

Briony is a 45-year-old housewife. Her only painless period was her first one, more than 30 years ago. Over the years, her pain had been treated in many ways, but never with lasting relief. Her first child was conceived easily, but she required IVF assistance for the second. After years of severely painful periods, often requiring pethidine injections, she was completely worn out by pain. We talked about the options:

- Do nothing and hope that menopause brought relief soon.
- Have a laparoscopy to remove any remaining endometriosis. This would improve the part of her pain due to endometriosis but not pain from the uterus itself.
- Six months of danazol or a GnRH analogue medication. This was unlikely to provide long-term relief, but would improve her pain for six to twelve months.
- A laparoscopic hysterectomy, with removal of any endometriosis present, but conservation of her ovaries.
- Investigation of complementary therapies.

Briony chose a hysterectomy. She was sick of the pain, and sick of the effect her pain had on her family. Some old endometriosis was found over one ureter. Her previous surgeon had left this area of endometriosis alone, due to its difficult location. Her pelvis was otherwise normal. The endometriosis was removed, and sent to pathology. The pathologist found adenomyosis too (see Chapter 9, page 151). Her pain had evolved over the years from prostaglandin and endometriosis pain as a young woman, through to old endometriosis and adenomyosis pain. Either way, it was all gone, and she was relieved. Briony described the operation pain as no worse than a period, but unlike a period, this pain would not come again.

Should my ovaries be removed?

In most cases, no.

Ovaries are important organs. They make hormones for wellbeing, and eggs for pregnancy. If your ovaries are healthy and you are not close to menopause then they should be kept, unless there are good reasons to remove them.

In the past, it was common for gynaecologists to recommend removal of both ovaries in woman with even mild endometriosis, to bring on an early menopause. It was hoped that this would cure her endometriosis. The endometriosis itself was left behind, but it was thought that the low oestrogen levels of menopause would remove the endometriosis without surgery. This type of treatment is now much less common.

Removing the ovaries worked for some women, but sometimes caused more problems than it solved. The areas of endometriosis left behind sometimes continued to cause pain, and the symptoms of early menopause (low oestrogen hormones) were often severe. When oestrogen hormone medications were taken to help the menopause symptoms, the endometriosis left behind often became active again, and the pain returned.

It is now almost always possible to remove endometriosis from an ovary without removing it. The ovary is 'repaired'. Repairing the ovary means removing the endometriosis and conserving as much of the ovary as possible. Small areas of endometriosis on the surface of the ovary can be cauterised. Chocolate cysts (Figure 5.2, page 45) inside the ovary can be removed with an operation called a *cystectomy*, and adhesions around the ovary can be divided. However, this surgery may be very technically challenging, and sometimes the endometriosis recurs.

Removing one or both ovaries, if they are seriously affected by endometriosis or adhesions, decreases the chance that you will need more surgery in the future, but can affect your fertility, and cause an earlier menopause. If only one ovary is removed, the other will take over the job of both ovaries, but if both ovaries are removed menopause will occur.

Whether or not your ovaries should be repaired or removed depends on several factors including your age, your plans for future pregnancy, and your personal preference. There are advantages and disadvantages with both treatment plans.

However, if your ovaries *are* to be removed, then the endometriosis should be removed too. You can then use the hormonal medications that you (as a young woman) need to feel well, with a lower chance that the endometriosis will recur. Once you reach the normal age of menopause (45 years of age or older), you can decide whether or not to continue your hormonal therapy, just as women who have never had endometriosis do.

Every woman's situation is different, but this is a guide to how I manage decisions about ovaries in my practice:

A young woman having her first laparoscopy

A young woman not only needs her hormones, but also does not know what her future plans for pregnancy may be. Personally, I never remove an ovary in a young woman at her first laparoscopy. I am usually able to remove all her endometriosis, with a cystectomy if necessary. If I am unable to treat all her endometriosis myself, I will remove those areas I can treat completely. If necessary, I will arrange a second laparoscopy performed together with a bowel or bladder surgeon. I do not remove ovaries in young women who are not expecting to have their ovaries removed.

A woman less than around 35 years of age, who has had a laparoscopy before and knows that she has severe endometriosis affecting her ovaries — or a woman over 35 who plans future pregnancies

The ovary can almost always be conserved, but this type of surgery requires specialised laparoscopic surgical skills. I always try to conserve as much normal ovary as possible. Occasionally, there are women whose pain is unlikely to improve without removal of a very severely damaged ovary. If so, after careful discussion, she may decide that the most severely affected ovary should be removed, and the least affected ovary be conserved. However, this is quite uncommon. Young women need their ovaries.

Before removing an ovary, I need to be sure that there is no other useful option available, that her pain is truly coming from that ovary, and that other causes of pain have been excluded. Remember that endometriosis is not a life-threatening condition, so there is time to consider what you want done.

A woman of approximately 35 to 45 years of age, with no future plans for pregnancy

Where healthy, I believe that the ovaries should still be conserved. They will provide hormones until menopause.

However, when the ovaries are seriously damaged by endometriosis or adhesions, I will occasionally remove one ovary if she has explained beforehand that she would be happy with this choice.

Some women are happy to leave the decision on whether or not to remove one ovary (if damaged) to my judgement at the time. Neither she nor I know exactly what will be found during her operation. We agree that I will not remove either ovary if they look healthy, but that if they are badly damaged by endometriosis, scar tissue or adhesions, I may remove one of them. I will repair and conserve the better of the two ovaries, and remove the one that looks most damaged. I will, of course, remove any other areas of endometriosis present, wherever possible.

Some women want both ovaries kept, regardless of whether or not they are severely damaged while others want both ovaries removed even if they look normal. They may have suffered repeated ovarian cysts or have cancer of the ovary in their family. It is always a question of balancing the different priorities.

A woman over 45 years of age

As normal menopause usually occurs between the ages of 45 and 55 years, removing the ovaries in this age group, and therefore hastening menopause, is less important from a medical point of view. Of course it may still be important for her body image. If a laparoscopy is needed, some women *choose* to have their ovaries removed, even if they look healthy, to decrease the chance of developing cancer of the ovaries in later life (see Chapter 8, page 136). This is a personal choice. If both ovaries are removed, then hot flushes usually start within a few days. Hormone replacement therapy (HRT) is available, if desired, to treat these symptoms.

A woman who is already past menopause

The ovaries are now no longer making oestrogen hormone. Few women in this age group need a laparoscopy, but if they do I offer to remove their ovaries to decrease the risk of ovarian cancer in later life.

It is important to be sure *before* your laparoscopy, that both you and your gynaecologist understand what surgery will be done if severe endometriosis involving the ovaries is found.

No matter how damaged they are, whether or not an ovary is removed remains your choice. Different women make different decisions. This is why it is important that your doctor knows what your preferences are before your surgery begins.

Will menopause cure my endometriosis?

No, but your symptoms should improve.

After menopause, when oestrogen levels fall, endometriosis usually becomes much less active. If your main problem has been period pain, you will probably find menopause a relief. Other symptoms associated with a normal monthly cycle such as menstrual migraine, hormonal mood swings and premenstrual syndrome should also resolve.

However, occasionally endometriosis does cause troublesome symptoms after menopause, even in women who do not use hormone replacement therapy. Scar tissue can affect nearby organs such as the ureter or bowel.

Using oestrogen replacement therapy (HRT) after menopause can stimulate any endometriosis that remains to become active again and cause symptoms. Your body likes the oestrogen replacement, but so does the endometriosis! This does not always happen, but it can make whether or not to use HRT an even more difficult decision than usual.

If your menopausal symptoms are severe, you may choose to start HRT, but stop it if your pains return. If you are already on HRT, it may be worthwhile reviewing it with your general practitioner every year or so, to see if a lower dose would be enough for you.

Endometriosis blocking the ureter after menopause

Katherine is a 53-year-old mother of three grown-up children a few years past menopause. In her forties a hysterectomy for heavy but not painful periods had been unexpectedly difficult. Her gynaecologist found many adhesions throughout her pelvis for which no cause was known. Several years later, Katherine developed pain on the right side of her pelvis. Katherine rarely complained, but this pain had been difficult to cope with. A laparoscopy showed that the right ovary was very firmly stuck to the side wall of the pelvis, just where the ureter lies. A large part of the right ovary was removed, but a piece that lay over the ureter was left to avoid damaging the ureter. Review of this tissue by a pathologist showed it to be endometriosis. We now had a reason for the scar tissue found at her hysterectomy many years before. Katherine had had severe endometriosis without pain, without any effect on her fertility and without realising it.

The pain on her right side improved for a few months, but then returned, higher up, near the kidney. An investigation called an IVP showed that the ureter on her right side was partially blocked. Urine could not pass easily from the kidney to the bladder. Katherine had another laparoscopy, this time with a kidney doctor (urologist) present to help. The blockage was caused by the remaining piece of scarred ovary pushing on the ureter. The rest of the ovary and all the surrounding scar tissue were removed through the laparoscope and her pain went away. We thought that would be the end of her problems, but a year later, the pain was back and another IVP showed that the ureter was again blocked. An operation through a large cut removed a golf-ball-sized amount of endometriosis from over the ureter and the ureter was re-attached to the bladder in a different position. Katherine has stopped her HRT to decrease the chance of more endometriosis. Will it come back again?

We don't know.

J have had a hysterectomy for endometriosis. What is the best form of HRT for me?

There is no one 'right' answer to this question, so I will explain what the issues are.

Most women on HRT take two hormones: an oestrogen that makes them feel well and a progestogen that protects the uterus from cancer. After a hysterectomy, the uterus no longer needs protecting, so taking a progestogen becomes unnecessary. Oestrogen can be taken by itself. This 'oestrogen-only HRT' is very popular as it is the progestogen that makes some women feel 'premenstrual' and the progestogen that may increase the risk of heart disease and breast cancer. So, for most women who choose to take HRT after a hysterectomy, including those with mild endometriosis, an oestrogen without a progestogen is probably the best choice.

The difficulty comes in women who have had severe endometriosis in the past, especially those whose endometriosis has not been removed. Taking oestrogen without a progestogen *might* increase the chance that the endometriosis becomes active again after menopause and *might* increase the small chance of cancer in the endometriosis that remains. Then again, it might not. Until we know more about how endometriosis responds to both these hormones, it is impossible to say what is the best HRT for women who have had severe endometriosis after hysterectomy.

Will my endometriosis become cancer?

Usually, no. Endometriosis is a benign condition, which means that it is not a cancer. So, for almost all women, the answer is *'No'*.

However, there are two less common types of ovarian cancer that are more common in women with endometriosis. These two types of cancer are called 'endometrioid' and 'clear cell' cancers. The words 'endometrioid' and 'clear cell' describe what the cancers look like under a microscope.

If these cancers are found, it may be impossible to know whether the cancer started in an area of endometriosis, in the ovary, or in the peritoneum near the ovary. As these cancers usually develop in older women, it has usually been many years between the diagnosis of endometriosis and the diagnosis of ovarian cancer. This is one reason why it is has taken such a long time for doctors to realise that there is any link between endometriosis and ovarian cancer at all.

Although this information is disturbing for women with endometriosis, it is not all bad news. Developing cancer in an area of endometriosis is still unlikely, and, cancers that do form in an area of endometriosis have a higher survival rate than other ovarian cancers.

Cancer of the ovary is difficult to diagnose as there are no good screening tests for it, and it usually causes few symptoms until it is quite advanced. This is why some older women who are having pelvic surgery (for whatever reason) sometimes choose to have their ovaries removed at the same time, even if the ovaries are normal. Removing the ovaries does not completely remove the risk of cancer, but it does make it much less likely.

How common is cancer of the ovary?

In Western countries, approximately 1 in 70 women develop cancer of the ovary during their lifetime. However, this risk may be around 1 in 40 for women with severe endometriosis affecting their ovaries (see References 18 and 19).

The risk of ovarian cancer is also increased in women with a close family history of ovarian or breast cancer. Some of these women have a particular genetic abnormality found on blood testing. Women with this type of genetic abnormality sometimes choose to have both ovaries removed once they have completed their family to decrease their risk.

What happens if cancer is found at my laparoscopy?

In rare cases, a woman having a laparoscopy for what is thought to be a benign (not cancerous) cyst is found to have what looks like a cancer. The gynaecologist must then decide what surgery to do. In my practice, if abnormalities are found which could be a cancer, I choose to take a biopsy (very small piece) of the abnormal area for a pathologist to check under a microscope, and do no further surgery that day. My patient wakes up having had a very short laparoscopy, from which she recovers quickly. We wait for the pathologist to decide whether or not it truly is a cancer, and if so, what type it is. If it is a cancer, then depending on what it is, the appropriate treatment is offered and the woman can contribute to the decision making herself.

Cancer in an area of endometriosis

Elizabeth is a 59-year-old teacher who had a hysterectomy and removal of both ovaries 20 years ago for management of her endometriosis. Her gynaecologist planned to remove both ovaries and any endometriosis, but there were so many adhesions present, and her operation was so difficult, that a small piece of ovary with some endometriosis was left behind on the left side.

Twenty years later, Elizabeth noticed a pain in her back on the left. She thought it was backache, but a scan of her spine looking for arthritis found a 7 cm lump in the left side of her pelvis.

The lump was removed and found to be an 'endometrioid'

type of ovarian cancer. There was no evidence of any cancer spread at her operation. Whether the cancer developed in an area of old endometriosis or in the small piece of remaining ovary is impossible to tell. Elizabeth had chemotherapy, which she tolerated well, and has returned to teaching. She is well.

What about complementary therapies?

Many women ask me this question. I have no training, nor experience, in complementary therapies so my opinions are those of a scientifically trained person who knows that modern medicine does not have all the answers, and remains open to new treatment options. This is why I am so pleased that Dr Margaret Taylor, a very experienced complementary therapist, has written Chapter 12.

Many of my patients tell me of the benefits they notice with complementary therapies, especially with regard to the hormonal changes they notice during the month. I am pleased for them, and happy with their choice. However, I feel nervous about recommending things I do not understand, so leave advice on these options to their natural therapist.

Do I think complementary therapies work?

Just like surgery and the medications that I might prescribe, I think they work for some women and for some problems. Complementary therapists see women for whom modern medicine has failed, and I see women for whom complementary therapies have failed. By working together, there is a good chance we can help most women. At our clinic we offer surgery, medications, counselling, lifestyle advice and links to complementary therapists we feel comfortable with.

For a doctor to say that any treatment 'works', we are required to have 'proof'. What does 'proof' mean? It means different things to different people, but I will try to explain what it means to a doctor.

Basically it means that large, well-designed trials have proven that the treatment is both safe and effective. In medicine we have been through times when it was enough for one or more doctors working with a medication to say that they thought it worked. This is no longer acceptable for medical treatments. Trials investigating the old claims have shown some to be true and others false. The improved knowledge the trials have provided has allowed us to move forward to better and more effective treatments over time.

Trials of any treatment usually divide a group of women into two groups. Half the women are given the herbal (or other) treatment and half are given a dummy treatment that looks the same (called a placebo). Neither group knows whether they are taking the real treatment or the dummy treatment. At the end of the treatment period, the number of women who feel better (or have had side effects) in each group are compared. The more women involved in the trial, and the more carefully the trial is run, the more reliable it is likely to be. Using a dummy tablet (placebo), allows for the fact that some women will get better by themselves over time with no treatment at all.

Trials such as these also look for side effects and safety issues for any treatment. If a herbal therapy can change the body enough to improve health, then it may also be able to cause side effects, even if these only affect very few people. To believe otherwise seems naïve, especially as throughout history some herbs have been used as poisons.

Have any herbal trials been done so far?

Yes. More and more herbal and diet therapy trials are being done, although as yet few involve treatments for endometriosis. These trials have shown a mixture of results. Some have shown clearly that herbal treatments are both effective and safe. For example, the nausea of pregnancy *is* less in women who use ginger supplements.

The symptoms of arthritis *are* improved with glucosamine. Cranberry juice *has* been shown to decrease urinary tract infections and evening primrose oil *can* improve sore breasts.

Other trials have shown no benefit for some treatments. For example, a Chinese herbal formulation was found to be no more effective than placebo for the hot flushes of menopause (see Reference 20).

What is more concerning is that some herbs have been linked to serious illness. For example, lead poisoning has been reported after the use of Ayurvedic (Indian) herbs; and black cohosh, despite its widespread use, has been associated with severe liver damage in very rare cases.

This is why the advice of an experienced herbal therapist is so important. For now, it is the personal advice of your herbal therapist and the quality of the place they source their herbs from that you will be relying on. The value of the care you receive will depend on their expertise and commitment to continued learning.

Whether it is surgery, medications or complementary therapies, we must all be honest with women about what we can and cannot achieve for them. If complementary therapies can improve our success in managing pelvic pain, then whatever they are, they are welcome. I look forward to any new ideas that improve the suffering of women with endometriosis. However, proof of effectiveness and information about side effects is the standard we should expect from whatever health care we choose. The challenge for complementary therapists is to work out which treatments (or combination of treatments) are truly effective and which are not, just as we have done in medicine. Once proven, these treatments will be rapidly accepted just as cranberry juice and glucosamine have been.

Over the next few years, the management of endometriosis will continue to change. New options for treatment will emerge and others will lose favour. Some of these new treatments may well come from areas considered as alternative today.

Which complementary therapies do I prefer?

As a scientifically trained person, before I can accept a new treatment, I need to understand how it *might* work, even if few details are available now. As I believe herbal therapies to be medications, I find it easy to accept that some herbal therapies do help endometriosis and the pain it causes. Equally, acupuncture and dietary therapy are based on sound principles. However, I find it very difficult to see any logical basis for homeopathy, where ingredients are diluted so extensively that no original product remains.

Then again, I have many friends (all dedicated to their homeopathic remedies) who will laugh at me for saying this!

Chapter 9

. . . .

What else could the pain be?

NOT ALL PERIOD OR PELVIC PAIN is endometriosis. Some women realise this when their laparoscopy shows a normal-looking pelvis with no endometriosis, and they are left wondering what to do about their pain. Their pelvis may *look* normal but it still hurts!

Others realise it after their endometriosis has been removed. Some of their symptoms improve, while others do not. Endometriosis was only one of their problems.

It is now time to look at other causes for your pain. Although these are common, you are now in a difficult position. Some of these conditions have only recently been shown to cause pain. Medical knowledge on how best to diagnose and treat them is improving, but is not yet complete.

In addition, no area of medicine covers all the possible conditions you may have, so there is no single professional who can offer everything you need. Some women spend years looking for the cause of their pain and a way to manage it. Distressingly, many never find the answers they need.

I suggest that this is where *you* may be able to help yourself. Each of the common causes of pelvic pain has its own fairly distinctive features. You are the one living with your symptoms every day, so with some information on what to look for, *you* may be able to work out what the problems are more quickly than your doctor can. You can at least bring up possibilities for discussion.

Recognising your pain from among those described in this chapter may point you in the right direction for the help you need, always bearing in mind that not every woman fits the normal picture for each condition. Once you have an idea about what your problem may be, then your general practitioner is the person who can help you put together a plan. Your general practitioner knows what services are available in your area. They can also help if your symptoms don't quite fit anywhere.

When thinking about your pain, consider what time of the month you get the pain, what makes it better, and what makes it worse. Your pain might be *cyclical*, which means that it occurs each month at a particular time of your menstrual cycle. Ovulation pain or period pain fit this pattern. Alternatively, your pain may be *chronic*, which means that it is long-term pain present on most days of the month. Remember that you may have more than one cause for your pain.

Some examples

Women with severe *period* pain after their endometriosis has been completely removed might have prostaglandin pain, adenomyosis, clot colic or pelvic congestion syndrome. None of these conditions show at a laparoscopy.

A woman with *chronic* pain after her endometriosis has been completely removed might have adenomyosis, neuropathic pain, interstitial cystitis, irritable bowel syndrome, adhesions, a pelvic infection or a mixture of these.

A woman with pelvic pain *after* a hysterectomy and removal of both ovaries might have neuropathic pain, more endometriosis, adhesions, interstitial cystitis, an ovarian remnant, or bowel pain.

The causes of pain described in this chapter include:

1 Pain from the uterus — adenomyosis, prostaglandin pain and clot colic
2 Pain from the bowel — irritable bowel syndrome, bloating, food intolerance and constipation
3 Pain from adhesions
4 Pain from nerves — neuropathic pain
5 Pain from muscles or joints — myofascial pain
6 Pain from the bladder — interstitial cystitis
7 Pain from ovaries — ovulation pain, functional ovarian cysts and ovarian remnant syndrome.
8 Pain from veins — ovarian vein syndrome and pelvic congestion syndrome.
9 Pain from the appendix
10 Endosalpingiosis
11 Pelvic infections — pelvic inflammatory disease.

It is easier to understand the different types of pain if you understand how we feel pain and what *referred pain* is, so this is described first in the section 'How we feel pain'. This background information is especially useful if you have chronic pain.

Is my pain just stress? Am I just weak?

No. You will notice that stress was not included as a cause of pain. We all know that stress can worsen a pain that already exists, but it is rarely the cause of the pain. A headache when you are happy and rested is a headache. A headache after a bad day, when you are tired and unhappy is unbearable.

Almost everyone nowadays has stress of some kind. Stress is a part of being human, rather than a weakness that should be hidden or denied. A certain amount of stress is useful. It keeps us motivated and active. Stress becomes a problem when it becomes overwhelming or impossible to resolve. Women with endometriosis have many reasons to be stressed.

How we feel pain

Imagine your finger touching a hot stove. The nerves in your finger notice the pain quickly and send pain signals from your finger to the brain. To reach the brain, the pain signal travels along a nerve to a part of the spinal cord called the *dorsal horn*. It then travels along another nerve up the spinal cord to the brain. It is when the pain signal reaches the brain that we feel pain.

Whether or not you notice the pain depends on how strong the pain signals are. A burn hurts a lot. It sends strong pain signals up to the brain, which acts rapidly to move your finger away from the stove.

There are always calming signals coming down from the brain telling us to ignore unimportant sensations such as clothes against our skin, or the normal function of body organs. A burn hurts so much that it quickly overcomes these calming signals and we feel pain. The normal filling and emptying of the bladder is an example of a slower, less urgent type of pain.

We do not notice our bladders filling until they are reasonably full because of the calming 'ignore bladder' signals coming down from the brain. Once there are more 'full bladder' signals going up to the brain than 'ignore bladder' signals going down to the bladder, we realise it is time to empty our bladder, but know that there is no hurry to do so. If we are doing something interesting at the time, we can still ignore our bladder, at least for a while. As the bladder fills even more, it becomes increasingly difficult to ignore, and the urge to empty the bladder becomes even stronger.

If there is a urine infection in the bladder, it becomes more irritable and sends 'full bladder' signals up to the brain even when it is not very full. The calming 'ignore bladder' signals are overcome much earlier than normal and the urge to pass urine comes more quickly. Because of this, women with a urine infection go to the toilet more often than usual. Equally, if you are anxious, there are fewer calming 'ignore bladder' signals going down to the bladder and the need to pass urine also comes earlier. Most women need to go to the toilet more often if they are anxious.

This is a good example of the interplay of emotions and pain. Anxiety does not cause a full bladder, but means that we notice the full bladder more. This is true of any unpleasant sensation. Our brain is more able to ignore it when our general physical and emotional health is good, and we send more calming signals down from our brain to whatever part of the body is painful.

Referred pain

Referred pain is pain felt in one part of the body, when the cause of the pain lies somewhere else. Why does it happen?

The spinal cord is divided into levels, one for each segment of the spinal cord. These segments have a name according to their position on the spinal cord (cervical, thoracic, lumbar or sacral) and a number within that area. For example, the first level in the lumbar part of the spinal cord is called L1, and the second level in the sacral part is called S2.

At each level of the spinal cord, two nerves feed into the dorsal horn. One of these nerves comes from an area of skin or muscle, and the other nerve comes from an organ inside the body such as the uterus, heart or diaphragm. For example, at the 10th thoracic level (T10), the dorsal horn receives one nerve from an area of skin and muscle over the lower abdomen, and one nerve from the uterus.

If a pain signal passes through either one of the two nerves that enter the spinal cord, it spreads to the other nerve as well. The brain becomes confused and cannot decide where the pain came from. Was the pain from the skin and muscle, or was it from the organ inside the body? If the brain cannot decide, it feels pain in both places, or sometimes just in the area that is actually normal and pain free. Pain felt in the area that is normal is called 'referred pain'.

There are several examples of this. During a heart attack, many people feel pain in their chest (via the nerve from the heart) *and* pain down their left arm (via the nerve from the skin and muscles of the arm). Both these nerves go into the spinal cord at the same level. There is nothing wrong with the skin and muscle of the arm, but the brain is confused and feels pain in both areas.

Another example of referred pain is the shoulder pain some women get for a few days after a laparoscopy. There is a segment of the cervical spinal cord in the neck (C4) that receives nerves from both the diaphragm *and* an area of skin over the shoulder. If a small amount of the gas used during the laparoscopy settles near the diaphragm and irritates it, pain is felt just below the ribs where the diaphragm is, but also in the shoulder. There is nothing wrong with the shoulder but the brain becomes confused and feels pain in both places. Sometimes the pain is only felt in the shoulder. When the gas near the diaphragm disappears, both pains go away.

Levels T10, T11, T12, L1, and L2 of the spinal cord receive nerves from both the abdominal wall over the lower abdomen or thighs *and* the pelvic organs. This means that pain in an area of the abdominal wall can cause referred pain deep in the pelvis. Equally, a pain in the pelvis can cause referred pain in the muscle wall of the abdomen or the thighs.

Other types of pain

Whether we feel 'touch' or 'pain' depends on how strongly the nerves in an area are stimulated. Light stimulation is felt as touch, and strong stimulation felt as pain. When pain has been present for a long time, structural changes in the nerves can affect the way a nerve sends pain signals. Eventually even light touch becomes painful, as the nerves that notice pain become more sensitive. In the pelvis this means that sensations that are not usually painful, such as normal bowel function become painful. This process is called *allodynia*.

Long-term pain can also cause *hyperalgesia*. This means that things that have always been painful become even more painful. The nerves that carry pain signals send more signals than usual when something painful happens. Once again, this is due to structural changes in the nerves.

Severe pain can also cause *wind-up* pain. This means that pain signals coming into one part of the spinal cord spread to levels of the spinal cord above or below that level. The brain then finds it even more difficult to know where the pain is coming from. Several levels are involved and the pain spreads to a larger area than before. For pelvic pain, this means that pain sometimes spreads above the navel on days when the pelvic pain is severe.

Wind-up pain

Lesley is a 38-year-old woman from the country. She had always had painful periods, but things were getting worse. Lesley had pelvic pain on most days, but the first day of her period was particularly painful. On these days she had a burning pain above her navel as well as her normal pelvic pain. Lesley agreed that the higher pain only happened on the days that her pelvic pain was severe. Burning pain often means neuropathic pain (see page 177).

When Lesley had a laparoscopy, endometriosis was found in her pelvis, but her upper abdomen was normal. Yes, she had pain from the endometriosis in her pelvis, but when this was bad, the pain impulse spread to nearby areas of her spinal cord (wind-up pain) and she felt the pain above her navel as well. To manage her pain, Lesley will need treatment for her neuropathic pain as well as her endometriosis.

1 Pain from the uterus

Pain from the uterus itself is the reason why removing endometriosis from around the pelvis does not always help period pain. Women who expected all their period pain to go after their surgery are often disappointed. They (and possibly their doctor) did not understand that before their surgery they had two types of pain: endometriosis pain *and* uterine pain.

What sort of pain is uterine pain?

Uterine pain occurs on the first one or two days of a period. The uterus is a hollow organ made of muscle. When the muscle tightens (contracts) at period time, it causes a cramp-like pain that comes and goes every few minutes. Between these contractions there is little pain. The pain may be referred to the thighs (but not past the knee) or into the lower back when it is severe. Uterine pain is felt across a large area in the centre of the lower abdomen. If your pain is felt in one small area, or on one side of the pelvis then other causes for your pain are more likely.

Pain during the month is less common but possible. If it is uterine pain, then it should worsen as a period comes closer and go away in the week after your period.

Some women with bleeding between periods notice that

whenever they bleed, they get pain that feels like a period. As the lining of the uterus bleeds it stimulates the muscle of the uterus to contract, which sometimes causes pain. If the irregular bleeding from the uterus can be stopped, these pains usually improve.

> **There are three main causes of uterine pain: adenomyosis, prostaglandin pain and clot colic.**

Adenomyosis

Adenomyosis might be new to you. While many women have heard the word endometriosis, few know about adenomyosis even though the two conditions are similar. While endometriosis is lesions that look like the lining of the uterus lying *outside* the uterus, adenomyosis is lesions that look like the lining of the uterus lying in the *muscle wall* of the uterus (see Figure 1.1, page 6).

Just like endometriosis, women with adenomyosis have painful periods. Some have pain through the month that worsens as the period comes closer. Others have heavy periods or pain with intercourse. The uterus is often a little enlarged, and your doctor may have described this as 'bulky'. A uterus may be bulky for other reasons, but adenomyosis and a bulky uterus often go together.

Endometriosis usually forms during a woman's teens and twenties, while adenomyosis usually forms during her thirties and forties. However, like most things in medicine, this is not always true. Occasionally quite young women are found to have adenomyosis, and certainly older women can develop new endometriosis. If your symptoms are like endometriosis, but none is found, then adenomyosis is a possible cause for your pain. Remember that you could have both conditions.

How is adenomyosis diagnosed?

Adenomyosis is difficult to diagnose because it lies in the muscle wall of the uterus between the inside and outside surfaces.

- *A hysteroscopy* (an operation through the vagina to look at the inside lining of the uterus) is usually normal, but will occasionally show tiny gland openings.
- *A laparoscopy* to look at the outside surface of the uterus is usually normal too, but will occasionally show an uneven texture in a bulky uterus. The major benefit of a laparoscopy is to exclude other causes of pain such as endometriosis or adhesions.
- *An ultrasound scan* done using a probe in the vagina on a high quality ultrasound machine may show a pattern of mottling in the wall of the uterus that is described by doctors as a 'rain in the forest' appearance. Even so, most ultrasounds are normal. If the adenomyosis forms a round lump in one part of the muscle wall it is called an *adenomyoma* and may look like a fibroid (see Chapter 8, page 128).
- *Histology* is the only reliable way to diagnose adenomyosis. Histology means that a pathologist has checked the uterus with a microscope. As this is only possible once the uterus has been removed it means that some women decide to have a hysterectomy for their symptoms without knowing whether they actually have adenomyosis or not.

What can I do about my adenomyosis?

The treatment of adenomyosis depends on your priorities. Putting together the right treatment plan for you means thinking about all your symptoms, your plans for future pregnancy and your personal preference.

Possible treatment options include:

- *No treatment.* Adenomyosis is not life threatening, so any treatment is optional.
- *A levonorgestrel releasing intra-uterine device (IUD)* (see Chapter 6, page 77). This device makes periods lighter, and sometimes improves the pain. If, once inserted, it does not suit you, then your doctor can remove it.
- *Progestogen* tablets or a progestogen injection to stop periods (see Chapter 6, page 75).
- *Anti-prostaglandin medications* (see Chapter 6, page 63) for period pain.
- *Danazol* in a low dose of around 200 mg daily. This makes periods lighter and less painful but is not a long-term solution (see Chapter 6, page 82).
- *The Pill*, taken continuously to avoid periods (see Chapter 6, page 80). If you do use the Pill, then choose one that is low in oestrogen or with a slightly higher progestogen dose.
- *Laparoscopic surgery* to remove an adenomyoma. This is only suitable *if* the adenomyosis lies together in an easily found lump. The operation can be done through a laparoscope, but it is a much more difficult operation than a hysterectomy.
- *Natural therapies.* As described in Chapter 12, these aim to reduce oestrogen dominance to make the adenomyosis less active.
- *Hysterectomy.* Most women with adenomyosis are over 35 years of age. Many have no further plans for pregnancy, and may have other gynaecological problems such as fibroids (Chapter 8, page 128) or heavy periods. For these women a hysterectomy to remove the problem permanently is a common and very reasonable choice. Obviously this is not suitable for young women, or those planning a future pregnancy.

If you are very close to menopause, you may decide to wait. When menopause arrives your oestrogen levels will fall and any adenomyosis will probably become less active. For most women, their symptoms improve substantially at this time. Then again, if you choose to use HRT after menopause, your oestrogen levels will not fall, and the adenomyosis will enjoy the hormones just as much as the rest of your body.

Who can help me with adenomyosis?

* Your gynaecologist. All gynaecologists can insert an intra-uterine device, prescribe medications for you, or do a hysterectomy. However, it takes a skilled laparoscopic surgeon to remove an adenomyoma without doing a hysterectomy.
* Your general practitioner can prescribe medications for you and may be able to insert an intra-uterine device.
* A natural therapist may be able to help some of these symptoms if they have expertise in this area.

A levonorgestrel IUD for adenomyosis

Diane is a 34-year-old single woman who would love to have a baby one day. Her periods were painful and heavy. A laparoscopy showed no endometriosis but a larger than normal uterus. A high quality ultrasound showed some 'mottling' in the wall of her 'bulky' uterus. Adenomyosis was the most likely diagnosis. Diane had always felt sick on the Pill, and was definitely not ready for a hysterectomy. She decided to try a levonorgestrel-releasing IUD. Six months later her periods were light. The pain had improved too. Diane still used pain medications each month but was now confident that she could manage her pain. The IUD can be removed when she is ready to have a baby.

Adenomyosis and hysterectomy

Saskia is a 40-year-old mother of two, working in an engineering office. Looking back, she had been very unsympathetic to friends with painful periods. Periods were never a problem for her, and she couldn't see what all the fuss was about. However, over the last two or three years her periods had become both painful and heavy. The pain was now severe, and an unexpectedly heavy bleed during a meeting with her male colleagues had left her embarrassed. Adenomyosis seemed much more likely than endometriosis.

Saskia had completed her family. She wished to spend time with them, without the pain and inconvenience of her periods. She chose a hysterectomy with conservation of her ovaries. Her ovaries will continue to make hormones for her so no hormone replacement is needed, but she knows there will be no bleeding and no period pain.

Prostaglandin pain

Prostaglandins cause the cramp-like period pain that makes a teenager's life so difficult on the first day of her period. They cause pain in some older women too, especially if they have never had children.

If the prostaglandins affect the nearby bowel, there may be bowel cramps or diarrhoea. If they spread to the rest of the body they may cause fainting, a slight temperature or nausea. Prostaglandin pain is better on the Pill or normal period pain (anti-prostaglandin) medications.

Just as the lining of the uterus (endometrium) can make prostaglandins, so can endometriosis lesions. This may be one of the ways in which endometriosis causes pain.

How is prostaglandin pain diagnosed?

There is no special test for prostaglandin pain. Prostaglandins do not change the appearance of any pelvic organ, so there is nothing unusual to see on an ultrasound scan, a laparoscopy or a hysteroscopy. These investigations only exclude other conditions such as endometriosis, adhesions or ovarian cysts. No blood tests are helpful.

However, if you have pain on the first day of your period that improves or goes away with anti-prostaglandin medications then they are the likely cause.

Why were my periods painless for the first few years?

When a girl first starts her periods, they are usually irregular. This means that they come at unpredictable times. Her body is mature enough to have periods, but not mature enough to release an egg from the ovary each month (that is, ovulate). These irregular periods are called *anovulatory cycles*. Over the next one to four years, as her body matures further, she will begin to ovulate each month and change to *ovulatory cycles*.

Ovulatory cycles are more painful than anovulatory cycles because more prostaglandins are released. So, as a girl's body matures, her periods become more regular but also more painful. As the Pill stops ovulation in most women, it usually helps this pain.

There are some women who never develop a regular cycle. They ovulate some months, but not others. The months where an egg is released are painful, while other months have no pain.

What can I do about prostaglandin pain?
Some medications prevent prostaglandins being made, and so treat the cause of the pain. They include:

- *Anti-prostaglandin medications* (see Chapter 6, page 63). Anti-prostaglandin suppositories work better than tablets but must be prescribed by a doctor.

- *An oral contraceptive pill.* A Pill that is low in oestrogen but higher in progestogen is best for period pain. Using the contraceptive pill to skip periods (see Chapter 6, page 80) means fewer periods and less pain.

- *Progesterone only contraceptives.* Contraceptives that use only progestogens usually work well. These include the 'Mini-pill', Implanon, and Depo-Provera.

- *A progestogen releasing intra-uterine device* (see Chapter 6, page 77). This provides a progestogen directly to the uterus with only a small amount absorbed to the rest of your body.

- *Other pain tablets* such as paracetamol, codeine and Tramal. These do not treat the cause of the pain. They make your brain less conscious of it. Tablets that include doxylamine, such as Mersyndol are useful for night-time pain relief. They should not be taken during the day if you will be driving or operating machinery in case they make you sleepy.

- *Acupuncture.*

Although having a baby does help some women with prostaglandin pain, there are other treatments for prostaglandin pain, and there is no guarantee that your pain would improve.

Fainting and severe pain once periods became regular

Ashleigh is a thin, fine boned, 19-year-old dancer. She had her first period at 14, and for two years her periods were irregular but not painful. Once her body matured and she began to ovulate each month, she suffered severe period pain especially on the day that bleeding began. The pain came suddenly, with little warning. With the pain came fainting so severe, that twice strangers had to call an ambulance when she collapsed.

> Ashleigh felt sure she must have endometriosis but a laparoscopy showed a normal pelvis. Although relieved that her pelvis was normal, her 'prostaglandin pain' needed management. Anti-prostaglandin medications work best if taken 12 to 24 hours before the pain starts and continued until the pain has settled. Ashleigh felt unable to time this reliably, so decided to use the Pill and have periods only every three months. This at least cut down the number of periods per year from twelve to four. Using the Pill, she could plan when her period would be, and take her anti-prostaglandin medications at the right time.

Who can help me with prostaglandin pain?

- Your general practitioner.
- A gynaecologist.
- An acupuncturist if they have expertise in this area.
- A natural therapist if they have expertise in this area.

Clot colic

Clot colic is a special type of period pain found in women with *heavy periods*. With the heavy bleeding come clots of blood and cramp-like pains. Once a clot is passed the pain improves, just as the pain of labour goes away once a baby is born. Clot colic only happens on the days you have clots. Pain on days when you bleed lightly is not clot colic.

A similar type of pain that is much *less* common can occur in women with a very narrow opening through their cervix. This is called *cervical stenosis*. Menstrual blood cannot pass through to the vagina easily and the uterus contracts forcefully to push it out.

What can I do about clot colic?

Any treatment that makes periods lighter will help clot colic.

In the past, women with heavy periods had few choices. Once their family was complete, many had a hysterectomy to solve the problem. Hysterectomy is still an option for women who have no future plans for pregnancy, but your gynaecologist now has other options to offer you. These newer techniques include:

- *Tranexamic acid.* This tablet is only taken during the heavy days of your period. It makes periods lighter by closing some of the blood vessels in the uterus, preventing them from losing as much blood. The best dose varies — 2 tablets, taken 4 times daily on the heavy days of your period gives the best results, but can make some women feel nauseous. A lower dose of 1 tablet 3 times daily is better tolerated if nausea is a problem. Women with a history (or family history) of blood clots in the legs or lungs should not take this medication.
- *A levonorgestrel-releasing intrauterine device (IUD)* (see Chapter 6, page 77). This releases a small dose of progestogen medication to the lining of the uterus every day. This thins the lining of the uterus making it less able to bleed. It can be removed later if you wish to become pregnant.
- *The contraceptive pill.* This makes periods lighter.
- *An endometrial ablation.* This operation destroys the lining of the uterus, making it less able to bleed during a period. It is *not* suitable for women who wish to become pregnant in the future.

Who can help me with clot colic?

- Your general practitioner.
- Your gynaecologist.

2 Pain from the bowel

There are many causes of bowel pain, but the commonest are irritable bowel syndrome (IBS), bloating, food intolerance and constipation.

What type of pain is bowel pain?

The bowel is a hollow muscular organ (like the uterus), so one type of bowel pain is a cramp-like pain that comes at regular intervals. The bowel contracts forcefully, much as it does if you have diarrhoea. If it is the lower bowel (called large bowel) that is affected, then the pain is felt below the navel. If it is the upper bowel (called small bowel) that is affected, then the pain is felt around the navel or sometimes above it.

Another type of bowel pain is a constant aching pain, often in the lower left side of the abdomen (near sections of bowel called the *sigmoid colon* or *rectum*), or in the lower right side of the abdomen (near a section of the bowel called the *caecum*). These types of pain are especially common in women with constipation. This type of pain is easy to confuse with ovarian pain, adhesions or endometriosis.

The most typical feature of bowel pain is that the pain improves once a bowel action has been passed. There are usually other bowel symptoms too, which might include diarrhoea, constipation, a need to strain to open your bowels, a feeling that the bowel is never empty, an urgency to use your bowels, the passage of mucus from the bowel, excessive wind or bloating.

Bowel pain occurs at any time of the month, not just with periods, but some women do find that their bowel symptoms are worse before a period.

Irritable bowel syndrome (IBS)

You may have already realised that IBS and endometriosis are easy to confuse. They cause similar pain in similar places. Many women who thought for years that their pain was due to an irritable bowel get better once the endometriosis they never knew they had is removed. Others who thought that all their symptoms were due to endometriosis feel much better once their IBS is treated.

IBS is a 'syndrome', which means that it is a collection of any of the bowel symptoms described above, all loosely put together under one name. Some women with IBS have a tendency to diarrhoea, while others tend to constipation. Very few women have all these symptoms, so your IBS symptoms may be different to those of your friends.

What causes IBS symptoms?

There is still a lot to learn about IBS, but it may be due to a change in how the nerves in the bowel work. Some of these nerves are 'motor' nerves that control how the bowel *moves*. A change in these nerves causes constipation, diarrhoea or a combination of the two. Other nerves are 'sensory' nerves that control how the bowel *feels*. A change in these nerves causes bloating, excess wind, a feeling that the bowel is never empty or urgency before the bowels are open.

Do some foods affect IBS?

Yes. For some women, there are particular foods that make their symptoms worse. Some of these foods are described on page 166. Other women never find a particular food to which they are sensitive, but know that eating a healthy, low fat, low salt, low caffeine and high fibre diet suits them best. This is, of course, the type of diet we should all eat for many reasons, not just our bowels. However, women with IBS respond to food in an exaggerated way, so while a large fatty meal can upset anyone's stomach, it will upset a woman with IBS more.

Even women without IBS often find that a healthy diet improves some aspects of their pelvic pain. If you have endometriosis, then the last thing you need is bowel pain too, so diet is important.

How is IBS diagnosed?

IBS is really common, so if you have any of these bowel symptoms then it is likely that at least *some* of your pain is due to IBS. However, before presuming that *all* your symptoms are IBS you should realise that it is what doctors call a 'diagnosis of exclusion'. This means that IBS can only be diagnosed after all other causes for the symptoms have been excluded. In young women, this may mean excluding endometriosis with a laparoscopy, or excluding other bowel conditions with blood tests, breath tests, X-rays, an endoscopy or a colonoscopy.

A laparoscopy cannot diagnose IBS as an irritable bowel looks the same as normal bowel through a laparoscope. Remember that many women have endometriosis *and* IBS.

What are a colonoscopy and an endoscopy?

The letters *-oscopy* in a medical word mean to have a look inside something with a telescope. A *lapar*oscopy means to look inside the abdomen and an *arthr*oscopy means to look inside a joint (often the knee). To check the bowel, a bowel doctor (gastroenterologist) uses slim, flexible telescopes. When they are passed through your mouth into the stomach and upper bowel, the procedure is called an *end*oscopy. When they are passed through the anus into the lower bowel, the procedure is called a flexible sigmoidoscopy or a *colon*oscopy. Both tests can be done with a light anaesthetic, so you need remember nothing and have no pain. Ask your doctor which technique they use.

Important symptoms to tell your doctor

Some symptoms should always be reported to your doctor straight-away. These include any bleeding from the bowel, bowel inconti-nence, getting up in the night to empty your bowels, unexplained weight loss, or malabsorption of food. Your doctor will also want to know if anyone in your close family has had bowel cancer.

Malabsorption of food means that food travels through your bowel without being digested properly. The bowel actions (faeces) are pale, smelly, and float. These are not the symptoms of irritable bowel, and may mean a serious bowel disorder. They need investigation.

Women over 50 hardly ever develop IBS for the first time, so if you are over 50 and your bowel habits have changed, you should see your doctor straight away. There are many innocent conditions that can cause this, but a cancer of the bowel needs to be excluded.

What can I do about IBS?

First, make sure that it actually *is* IBS:

- *Tell your doctor about any of the important symptoms above.*
- *Consider whether you could have coeliac disease, fructose intolerance or lactose intolerance.* See page 166.
- *Check your medications and herbal supplements.* Antibiotics, antacids, laxatives, thyroid supplements or some blood pres-sure tablets can worsen diarrhoea. Amitriptyline, iron tablets, painkillers, tranquillisers and other blood pressure tablets can worsen constipation. Many herbal therapies affect the bowel. Your doctor or herbal therapist may have an alternative medi-cation you can use.

Then try some of these suggestions. They won't all be right for you, but some will:

- *Lifestyle changes.* This means avoiding things that make your symptoms worse, like alcohol and stress. Eating regular meals in an unhurried way and getting enough sleep are good for your bowel. The nicotine in cigarettes irritates the bowel, so if you smoke, then now is always a good time to quit.

- *A better diet.* Just as you have more to lose from a bad diet than other women, you have more to gain from a good diet. Your bowel likes a healthy, low fat, low salt, low caffeine and high fibre diet.

- *Diet advice for particular symptoms.* If you have indigestion or burping, then avoid chocolate, alcohol or coffee. If you have an easily irritated stomach, then tomatoes, citrus fruits, alcohol, and spicy foods are best avoided.

- *Eat more fibre.* A Western diet rarely has enough fibre for our bowels. Most women (but not all) feel better eating more fibre, but you should start it slowly.

- *Care for your bowel bacteria.* It is the bacteria in our bowel that help us digest our food. Some foods contain live bacteria and may help some symptoms. However, there is still a lot to learn about which bacteria help which symptoms. These bacteria enjoy a high fibre diet so increasing the amount of fibre you eat will encourage them to work better for you.

- *Complementary therapies.* Herbal teas, and slippery elm are commonly used for IBS symptoms. Peppermint oil capsules taken 3 or 4 times daily half an hour before meals often help abdominal pain and bloating, but can aggravate indigestion.

- *Manage your stress.* This is an important part of your care. Stress aggravates IBS and bowel symptoms are particularly common in women who have suffered physical or sexual abuse in the past.

- *Medications.* Most women with IBS don't need medications. There is no medication that treats all the symptoms of IBS and no medication that will 'cure' IBS. The right medication for you will depend on your particular symptoms.

- Fibre supplements help constipation, bowel pain and sometimes diarrhoea.
- Antispasmodics such as mebeverine, or 'tricyclics' such as amitriptyline improve painful bowel contractions.
- Laxatives avoid constipation but are rarely necessary on a high fibre diet.
- Loperamide helps diarrhoea.
- Medications that treat the muscles and nerves of the bowel themselves include Tegaserod (if you tend to be constipated) and Allosetron (if you tend to get diarrhoea).

Some of these suggestions (lifestyle changes, a generally healthy diet and more fibre) will help almost anyone with bowel problems. Others (like checking for food allergies or intolerances) will only help some women. If possible, change only one or two things at a time, so you will know what helps you most.

Finally, you do not have to treat IBS. If your symptoms are mild, then maybe just making the diagnosis and knowing that it is nothing more serious is enough for you.

Why is IBS worse with stress?

No-one really knows why stress makes some IBS worse. However, the chemicals our brain makes when we are stressed are similar to some of the chemicals that affect the bowel. Stress chemicals may change the way our bowel moves or feels. It is also possible that stress chemicals alter the way our brain feels pain.

Food intolerance and food allergy

Could your diet be aggravating your bowel symptoms? Cutting out anything at all that could possibly affect you may help (at least in the short term), but we all need to eat. We also need to feed our families and eat the right food to keep our body healthy long term. By finding out which foods bother you most, which ones you can eat in small quantities and which ones cause you no problems at all, you can usually avoid excessively strict or restrictive diets.

There are two main ways that food can cause problems: food intolerance and food allergy.

Food intolerance means that the bowel cannot digest certain foods easily. Eating a little of a particular food may cause no problems at all, as the bowel can cope with small amounts. However, eating larger amounts of that food overloads the bowel and causes cramps, diarrhoea or bloating. The common causes of food intolerance are lactose (in milk products), and fructose (see page 167).

Food allergy means that the body's immune system reacts to a particular protein in a food. Sometimes the immune system reacts quickly causing a life-threatening condition called *anaphylaxis*, but usually it reacts slowly causing a variety of problems that may be hard to pick as a food allergy. The commonest foods to cause food allergy are milk, eggs, fish, nuts, shellfish, soybeans and gluten (wheat). Food allergies are less common than food intolerances.

Lactose intolerance
Women with lactose intolerance find it difficult to absorb foods containing lactose such as milk, cheese or ice cream. This is not a food allergy: the body just finds it hard to digest. Lactose intolerance can be diagnosed with a 'breath test' arranged by your general practitioner. If you are found to be lactose intolerant, it is important that you see a dietician for expert advice on how to cut down on milk, while still getting the calcium you need for your bones. Most women with lactose intolerance have mild symptoms that are easily treated by cutting down on how much milk, or milk products they eat at any one time.

Some people who have never shown food intolerance develop a type of lactose intolerance if they cut out lactose for a period of time. For example, Western people who travel to Asia and live on a traditional Asian diet (very low in milk products), then return home and drink a milkshake or eat a large amount of cheese should expect an upset bowel. They are not allergic to milk products, but until their body adjusts back to their old diet, they have temporary lactose intolerance.

Fructose intolerance

Fructose is a sugar found in fruit, but also found in food compounds called *fructans* that release fructose as they are digested. It is normal to absorb fructose slowly from the bowel but if you have a sensitive bowel, what is normal for other women may cause you to suffer bloating, pain or diarrhoea. This is not a food allergy. A small amount of fructose or fructan causes no problems at all, but a larger amount taken all at once is more than the bowel can cope with and diarrhoea, bloating or pain result.

Fruit is an important part of everyone's diet, so a fructose-free diet is not sensible. However, if you cut down on fruits or foods that are high in fructose, and replace them with fruits or foods that are low in fructose, you may suffer fewer bowel symptoms. Fructose is also absorbed more easily from the bowel if another sugar called 'glucose' has been eaten at the same meal.

- *Foods that are high in fructose or fructans include:* wheat-based products (bread, pasta, biscuits), onions, sucrose-sweetened fizzy drinks, apples, pears, honey, and corn syrup (a sweetener in some foods). These foods are best eaten in small quantities or spread across the day if you have an irritable bowel.
- *Foods that are low in fructose or fructans include:* bananas, apricots, plums, berries, oranges, lemons and glucose-sweetened fizzy drinks.

Coeliac disease

Around one in 200 people have coeliac disease. When they eat a protein called *gluten*, their body's immune system makes antibodies that attack their bowel. The damaged bowel can no longer absorb iron and vitamins from food. Gluten is found in wheat, rye and barley, but not in rice, corn or potatoes. Some coeliacs have weight loss and diarrhoea, so their condition is diagnosed when they are very young, but many coeliacs have few symptoms and it is found during investigation of an unexpectedly low iron level, or mild bowel complaints.

Nowadays most coeliac disease can be diagnosed with a blood test. The most reliable tests measure endomysial or transglutaminase antibodies. A test for gliadin antibodies is less reliable. While the blood tests are useful, if they are positive you may still need an endoscopy to be completely sure of the diagnosis. Remember that neither the blood tests, nor an endoscopy can diagnose coeliac disease if you have already cut gluten out of your diet, so it is very important to have the tests done *before* changing your diet.

What is the difference between coeliac disease and gluten intolerance?

There are many people, both men and women, who don't have coeliac disease but feel better on a low gluten or low wheat diet. These people are called 'gluten intolerant' although it may be that they feel better because their new diet is low in fructans rather than because it is low in gluten (see above). Certainly most women with bloating feel better when they cut down on bread, cakes and biscuits.

While people with coeliac disease should eat *no* gluten whatsoever for the rest of their life, a person with gluten intolerance (or fructan intolerance) can eat *small* amounts of gluten without problems.

Whatever food issues you have, a special diet is difficult to stick to, a lot of trouble and can be expensive. Then again, if it helps your symptoms then the effort may be worthwhile. If you do plan to cut down on lactose, fructose or gluten, a dietician can help you plan a diet that still provides the nutrients your body needs.

Bloating

Doctors often think of bloating as an inconvenience rather than a major problem. This is because bloating rarely means a serious illness, but also because it is poorly understood and there are no easy answers to the problem. But if you ask women about their bloating, they see it as a major problem: possibly their worst symptom. Bloating makes women feel unfeminine, unattractive and uncomfortable. It also makes any other pelvic pain worse.

So what is bloating?

There are two types of bloating:

- *Bloating where the abdomen swells due to excess wind.* This may be due to swallowing excess air when you talk or eat, or to certain foods in your diet. If your body can't absorb some foods, they stay in the bowel for longer. Bacteria in the bowel ferment these foods, making gas. Unless you have coeliac disease, you are not allergic to these foods, but you may need to eat them in smaller quantities.
- *Bloating where the abdomen looks normal, but feels bloated.* This is usually due to IBS. In women with IBS, the bowel does not move normally so wind doesn't pass through easily. The nerves in the bowel are hyper-sensitive so the bowel feels uncomfortable too. This type of bloating gets worse during the day and is best first thing in the morning.

What can I do about bloating?

We are all different and what causes you to bloat may cause your friend no problems at all. This list describes some of the problems that can cause bloating. It is very unlikely that they will all apply to you, but one or two of them may.

- *Are you swallowing too much air when you talk or eat?* This is more likely if you eat in a hurry, chew gum, drink fizzy drinks or smoke cigarettes. Chewing gum also contains sorbitol, a that causes bloating and diarrhoea.
- *Are you eating too much fructose or fructan?* (See page 167). Cutting down on floods with flour such as bread and biscuits often helps.
- *Are you wearing tight-waisted clothes or panty hose?* These make you feel more uncomfortable.
- *Do you spend a lot of your day sitting down?* A brisk walk at lunchtime will help the wind pass and your bowel work normally.
- *Do you eat a lot of fermenting vegetables?* It is normal for foods such as beans, lentils, brussels sprouts, cabbage and legumes to make gas during their digestion. They are not bad foods, but they do make gas.

So what can I eat?

We all need to eat. We all have lives to live as well. Very few of us have the time to spend finding special food or preparing compli-cated menus. If you are confused after reading all the dietary advice, remember that a simple healthy diet that is low fat, low sugar, low caffeine and high fibre will suit most women well. This diet is suitable for your family too.

Food should be enjoyed. While it is useful to look at foods and how they affect you, they should not rule your life. Even if you have a food intolerance, most women can still enjoy most of the foods they like, but in smaller quantities and not all at once. It is only when someone has a food allergy that it means a food should never be eaten.

Constipation

Almost no-one in Western countries eats enough fibre for their bowel to work well. Constipation is common. It causes a cramp-like pain that improves once the bowels have been opened well. Mild constipation may be one reason why a healthy diet improves some bowel pain. It treats the constipation no-one knew was there.

As well as eating a low fibre diet, many women do not place a high enough priority on their bowel function. Life is busy. Women tend to rush in, strain, and then if no bowel action occurs quickly, give up and hope something happens later in the day. They have lost an opportunity.

The best time to open your bowels is in the morning after breakfast because this is when the bowel contractions are strongest. They start while you are asleep — about an hour or so before your bowel actually opens.

These contractions begin high up in your bowel, move the bowel action around to the lower bowel and then out through the anus. They can open your bowels much more efficiently than you can by straining your pelvic floor muscles, but they do take time. Stress or anxiety can interfere with them — or with your awareness of the need to open your bowels. Straining is harmful to the pelvic floor and should not be necessary if you have a normal bowel, give them time and have enough fibre in your diet.

How can J increase the fibre in my diet?

There are two types of fibre: soluble fibre and *in*soluble fibre. Soluble fibre is found in fruits and grains. It is digested in the bowel, and keeps both the bowel wall and the bacteria in the bowel healthy. Insoluble fibre is found in the outside shell (husk) of grains. It holds water, makes your bowel action larger and helps food pass through the bowel faster.

You can increase the fibre in your diet by eating more high fibre food (multigrain breads, high fibre cereals, fruit etc.), or if necessary using a fibre supplement. Either way, you should always increase the fibre in your diet slowly to avoid bloating.

When starting a fibre supplement, start with 1 teaspoon each morning with plenty of water. This can be increased to 2 teaspoons daily after a week, and then 3 teaspoons daily, if necessary, a week later. Sterculia (Normafibe) causes less bloating than most other fibre supplements.

What can I do about my constipation?

Before seeing your doctor, there are several things you can do yourself:

- Eat enough fibre
- Eat breakfast every day
- Give yourself enough time to go to the toilet each morning
- Drink enough fluid. No fibre will work well unless you drink enough water. Two litres of fluid, mostly water, is best
- Do regular exercise such as brisk walking each day.

If you still have problems:

- Talk to your general practitioner about your general health. Low thyroid hormone levels can worsen constipation.
- Check the medications you use. Amitriptyline, strong pain medications, some tablets for mental health problems and the long-term use of strong laxatives can all slow the bowel.
- See a pelvic floor physiotherapist to improve your pelvic

muscle function and bowel habits.
- See a dietician to review your diet.
- See a bowel doctor (gastroenterologist) if your problems continue.

My constipation is very severe. Nothing works for me.

A small number of women have severe constipation even when they eat a high fibre diet. They suffer abdominal pain or bloating and use laxatives or enemas frequently. If this is you, then you should see a gastroenterologist. Severe constipation may be due to a very slow bowel or a bowel that is partly blocked. Special medical tests are needed to work out the cause of the problem and how best to treat it.

IBS, bloating, food intolerance and constipation are the problems that bother women with pelvic pain or endometriosis most, but there are others. If your symptoms change over time you should go back to your doctor to discuss them again. You may have developed a new condition, or what was thought to be irritable bowel syndrome may turn out to be something else. If you are unsure, your general practitioner or bowel doctor is the best person to see.

Who can help me with bowel pain?
- Your general practitioner.
- A bowel doctor (gastroenterologist).
- A dietician.
- A physiotherapist with a special interest in pelvic conditions if you have constipation or tight pelvic floor muscles.
- A natural therapist.

3 Pain from adhesions

You may have been told that there are adhesions in your pelvis. So what are adhesions? Adhesions are areas where organs have become stuck together. Just as an adhes*ive* is another name for a glue, an adhes*ion* means a point where organs have become 'glued' together (see Figure 2.1 on page 16). Adhesions can affect fertility if they are near the ovary or the fallopian tubes.

What sort of pain can adhesions cause?

Adhesions around an ovary cause pain felt on one side of the pelvis, that is particularly severe during ovulation. Ovaries are sensitive organs. They like to move freely (just like testes) and become painful if tied down by an adhesion. At ovulation, the ovary changes in size. There is more tension on the ovary at this time and the pain worsens. If the ovary is stretched even further by a 'functional cyst' (see page 195), then the pain becomes even more severe. As women who are on the Pill do not usually ovulate, they have less pain from adhesions affecting the ovary.

Adhesions in other areas of the pelvis are less likely to cause pain than ovarian adhesions. If they do cause pain, it is always felt in the same part of the pelvis. It may be worse with sudden movement or intercourse. A tender area in a pelvic muscle may cause a similar type of pain (see page 183).

Adhesions between loops of bowel rarely cause pain unless they block the bowel, or prevent normal bowel function.

What causes adhesions?

Anything that irritates the lining of the abdomen (peritoneum) can cause an adhesion. The common causes include endometriosis, a pelvic infection, an operation (especially if it is done through a large cut), or severe appendicitis where the appendix has ruptured. However, in some women, no cause for the adhesions can be found. If you have had pelvic surgery in the past, then you should expect that you have at least *some* adhesions, but as most adhesions do not cause pain, they may not require treatment.

How are adhesions diagnosed?

Unfortunately, only a laparoscopy will reliably show if you have adhesions, and whether or not they involve the ovary. Even women who have many reasons why they *might* have adhesions do not. Equally, some women have more adhesions found during a laparoscopy than expected. Adhesions do not show on an ultrasound scan.

Can adhesions affect my surgery?

Yes. Adhesions make any operation more difficult because:

- They block the surgeon's view of the pelvis through the laparoscope. Dividing the adhesions to allow a better view makes the operation longer.
- They may mean less room for the laparoscopic instruments. This makes the operation slower.
- Organs that are stuck together are more easily damaged when the adhesions are divided.
- They may hide important organs like the ureter under scar tissue. This makes them easier to damage during an operation.

For all these reasons, adhesions make the chance of a hole (perforation) in an organ higher than usual (see Chapter 5, page 55).

Can adhesions be prevented?

Sometimes, yes.

Safe sexual practices mean fewer sexually transmitted disease and less risk of pelvic infection. Treating endometriosis early and effectively may decrease the chance of adhesions. Surgery through a laparoscope, rather than a larger cut, is less likely to cause adhesions. This is one of the strengths of laparoscopic surgery. Gentle handling of tissues by your surgeon, and care to control any bleeding are important, and an adhesion barrier placed near the ovaries during surgery may keep them apart during the healing phase. There are many different types of adhesion barriers, but most dissolve over one or two weeks. None are perfect and none will avoid all adhesions, but they may make them less likely.

Unfortunately, one factor that cannot be changed is your own skin type. Some women have tissues that make lots of adhesions even after minor surgery. Others have many operations yet form few adhesions.

What can I do about the adhesions that I have?

- *Do nothing.* Adhesions only matter if they cause pain. No treatment may be necessary.
- *The contraceptive pill.* This helps ovulation pain because it prevents the ovary changing shape at ovulation.
- *A laparoscopy to divide the adhesions.* When the organs are loosely tied together, this is not difficult. The adhesions lie like fine curtains between the pelvic organs and are easily cut using scissors or laser (see Figure 2.1, page 16). However, dividing organs that are firmly fixed together is one of the most difficult areas of laparoscopic surgery. It is very easy to make a hole (perforation) in one of the organs involved. This hole then needs to be repaired. (See Eleanor's case study in Chapter 5, on page 55.)
- *Surgery to remove one or both ovaries.* This only applies to older women with completed families.

The difficulty with dividing adhesions is that even when separated beautifully, the adhesions often reform. This is less likely after a laparoscopy than a laparotomy but it can still happen.

Who can help me with adhesions?

- A laparoscopic surgeon (gynaecologist) if surgery is required. Almost all adhesions can be divided through the laparoscope, but not all gynaecologists perform this type of surgery.
- A dietician if your adhesions affect your bowel and he or she has a special interest in this area.
- Your general practitioner if you would like to use the contraceptive pill.

4 Pain from nerves – neuropathic pain

Neuropathic pain is different to other pain. The endometriosis is gone, no other problems have been found, but there is still pain. This is the pain described by women who say, 'Nothing seems to work for me.' Neuropathic pain is easier to understand if you have read about how we feel pain in Chapter 9, on page 146.

What type of pain is neuropathic pain?

Neuropathic pain is constant pain, not just pain with periods. It is present on most days. The pain may be burning, sharp, or stabbing. If it is the nerves of the abdominal wall that are affected, there may be a numbness or unusual feeling when that area is touched. Many normal activities such as moving, stretching, or opening your bowels cause pain. Neuropathic pain symptoms vary from day to day. It is a 'wearing' pain that often disturbs sleep.

Your abdomen may not *look* swollen, but *feels* swollen in the same way that your lip feels swollen after an anaesthetic at the dentist. This is especially common in women who have scars on their abdomen that are numb to touch. There may be allodynia, hyperalgesia or wind-up features to your pain (see page 149).

Women with neuropathic pain often wake up after an operation with no pain, overjoyed that their pain has gone. This is because the medications used by the anaesthetist to put you to sleep treat neuropathic pain very effectively. Unfortunately, the pain often returns over the next few weeks or months once the effect of the medication wears off.

What is neuropathic pain?

Neuropathic pain is pain that starts in the nerves themselves at some point on their pathway from the pelvis to the brain. For any one of many reasons, the nerve pathway from the pelvis to the brain has become 'sensitised' and well established. The nerves have learned to transmit pain very well, and cannot unlearn it. The original cause of pain may be gone, but the nerves are unable to forget the pain they knew before.

The idea of neuropathic pain as a cause of *pelvic* pain is fairly new, but it has been recognised as a cause of pain in other parts of the body for some time. Examples of this type of pain include nerve damage from a prolapsed intervertebral disc, diabetes or a genital herpes infection. For each of these conditions, the reason for the pain is different.

A prolapsed disc puts pressure on a nerve. Even when an operation takes pressure off the nerve, the nerve may remember the pain and continue to send pain signals. Long-term diabetes can chemically damage nerves, which then transmit pain. Men or women with genital herpes have small ulcers like cold sores on the scrotum or labia caused by the herpes virus. Over two weeks the ulcers heal completely but the pain may continue. In all these examples, a condition has injured, upset or irritated a nerve, and the nerve has continued to transmit pain even when the cause of the pain has gone. Endometriosis, surgery or long-term pain itself can all cause permanent structural changes to nerves.

What can I do about neuropathic pain?

Like endometriosis, it is only in the last ten years or so that much has been known about how to manage neuropathic pain effectively. This does not mean that treating neuropathic pain is easy, but there is much more available now.

Of the many ways of treating neuropathic pain it is unlikely that any one of these will magically provide a complete cure. Once chronic pain becomes established, it may be not be possible to eliminate it completely. The best results are achieved with a mix of medications, and lifestyle changes. The good thing is that even if your pain is not completely cured, you *can* expect a big improvement.

Medicines that can help neuropathic pain

The medicines used include:

- *Tricyclic medications* such as amitriptyline. These medications increase the calming signals sent down from the brain, so that fewer pain signals get through. (See Chapter 6, page 72).
- *Anti-convulsant medications* such as gabapentin, pregabalin and sodium valproate. Anticonvulsant medications are usually used to treat epilepsy. They stabilise the nerves and make them less irritable (See Chapter 6, page 74).
- *Anti-prostaglandin medications* taken regularly once daily. These improve the chemical environment around the nerves. They are best used in combination with either gabapentin, pregabalin or amitriptyline.
- *Tramadol.* Tramadol is an opioid medication, but it has other actions too.
- *Other medications* such as mexiletine, ketamine, magnesium, local anaesthetics or corticosteroids.

Normal pain medications such as codeine or pethidine do *not* work well for neuropathic pain. You may have worked this out already.

Treatments that don't involve taking medicines

- *Exercise.* Neuropathic pain feels better after rest because there is less activity in the nerves. However, long-term rest is a trap. You will have less pain if your body is fit and active. It is important that you see daily exercise and increased muscle strength as part of your pain management program. Don't do too much too soon. Start with gentle exercise that you can do easily (eg. walking), do it regularly and build up slowly. The endorphin chemicals made during exercise improve wellbeing too.

- *Maintain your interests.* This gives your brain other things to think about apart from your pain. Are there things that were important to you before your pain? Are there activities that you enjoy? Are there goals you *can* achieve despite your pain?

- *Get enough sleep at night.* Tired nerves are more irritable.

- *Avoid being overweight.* A heavier body weight overloads your muscles and joints. You do not need a new cause of pain (see page 183).

- *Manage your stress.* A relaxed brain sends more 'ignore pain' signals to balance your pain better.

Gabapentin for neuropathic pain

Isobel is a 35-year-old teacher whose severe endometriosis had been removed at an extensive laparoscopic operation by an experienced endometriosis surgeon a few years before. The endometriosis had been removed, but she still had pain that bothered her every day and often at night. She was worn out and worried that she just wasn't herself. When the pain was particularly severe in her pelvis, she felt pain above her navel too. This was 'wind-up' pain. She also suffered constipation, ovulation pain, and a pain in her **urethra**. Isobel no longer had endometriosis, but she certainly had several causes of pain.

Isobel started gabapentin to treat the part of her pain that was neuropathic. She described the first month on her treatment as 'liberating'. The pain above her navel and most of her pelvic pain had gone. She slept well. Her friends felt that they needed whatever had made her look so obviously well!

Gabapentin will not treat her ovulation pain, (due to adhesions around an ovary), her constipation pain, or her urethral pain (see page 189). They will need to be managed separately, but at least she now has the energy to work on her other pains. A doctor who uses medications to treat brain, spine and nerve conditions (neurologist) will continue the management of her neuropathic pain.

So which treatment mix is best for me?

Working out the best combination of these treatments for your pain may be too difficult for your gynaecologist.

The following combination of treatments will help most women:

- One of amitriptyline, gabapentin or pregabalin, with
- One of ibuprofen, diclofenac or naproxen with food once daily, with
- Regular exercise and regular sleep, with
- A healthy diet

Fortunately, if you need more help there are now pain specialists who manage a wide variety of chronic pain conditions in both men and women. Pelvic pain is just one of the conditions they see. Such specialists work in 'pain clinics' and have a lot to offer. If you have neuropathic pain, a pain specialist is the best person to advise you on which mix of treatments will suit you best.

Before going to a pain clinic, it is important that any endometriosis lesions have been completely removed. Pain clinics do well for women with neuropathic pain, but are less successful if you still have endometriosis present. If it has been a long time since your last operation, it may take another laparoscopy to be sure that other causes of pain have been excluded.

A pain clinic uses what is called a multi-disciplinary approach to pain management. This means that professionals from many areas of medicine work together to get the best result possible for each individual person. The pain clinic team might include doctors (a pain specialist, an anaesthetist, a psychiatrist and a rehabilitation specialist), as well as physiotherapists, occupational therapists, psychologists and others. It is this mix of skills that makes pain clinics so successful. If you go to a pain clinic, it is unlikely that you will see all of these people, but they are there if needed.

As most women with endometriosis have been told at one time (or many times) that their pain was psychological, it is not surprising that some are suspicious when asked to see the psychologist or psychiatrist who works in the pain clinic. There is no need to be. If your pain specialist recommends psychological help it is not because they think your pain is imaginary. It is because your recovery will be slower if you are stressed, depressed or anxious.

The only good thing about neuropathic pain is that treatments are improving. What was once almost untreatable is now manageable. However, it will take effort on your part, a mixture of treatments and good advice.

Who can help me with neuropathic pain?
- A pain clinic gives the most complete care.
- Your general practitioner.
- Your gynaecologist may be happy to prescribe some of these medications if he or she has an interest in this area.
- A neurologist.

5 Pain from muscles or joints – myofascial pain

Muscle pain is not something many women think of when they have pelvic pain. Tender points in the neck and shoulders have been known about since the 1940s, but it is only recently that similar points in pelvic muscles have been recognised as a common cause of pelvic pain in women.

These tender points cause pain that feels as if it comes from the pelvic organs (uterus, ovaries, bladder or bowel). This is because the nerves that carry pain signals from the muscles of the abdomen, back, thighs or pelvis join the nerves that carry pain signals from the pelvic organs when they reach the spinal cord, and before they reach the brain.

What type of pain is muscle or joint pain?

Muscular pain is described as dull, aching or deep pain. It is worse on some days than others, but felt on most days. It may be aggravated by changes in position, and made either better or worse with exercise. Muscle or joint pain is difficult to diagnose because it is often 'referred' to other areas of the pelvis. Some examples of this include:

- A tender point in the muscle of the abdominal wall on one side felt as pain coming from the ovary on that side. The ovary itself is normal.
- A tender point in the muscles of the lower back felt as pain in the uterus or bladder. The uterus and bladder are normal. Other lower back conditions such as a prolapsed disc or strained ligaments cause a similar pain.
- The pain from a cut in the abdomen after an operation referred to pain in the pelvis.
- Tender points in the muscles of the inner thigh referred to the

vagina. This pain is worse if the thighs are spread apart, making some sexual positions painful.

- Tender points in the muscles lining the pelvic bones, causing pain that seems to come from the uterus or ovaries.
- Tender, over-active pelvic floor muscles causing pelvic pain and painful sex.

How can I tell if I have muscle or joint pain?

There is no blood test or scan that can prove your pain is muscular. It is diagnosed from your description of the pain, and the finding of tender spots during a physical examination that when pressed cause your particular pain. Joint pain is uncommon in young women, but can be investigated with an X-ray, or CT scan if it seems likely.

Think about when you get your pain. Is the pain worse in some positions, after certain movements or with exercise? If so, then at least part of the pain may be muscular. A 'pain diary' is useful. Episodes of pain are written down each day, together with your other activities, any emotional stress and the stage of your menstrual cycle. Over time, a pattern of pain at certain times or with certain activities may become obvious.

Muscle or joint pain is especially common if:

- You have injured your back, pelvis or knees.
- You have problems with posture, such as a lordosis ('sway back'), a scoliosis (curved spine), a short leg, a stiff or unstable sacroiliac joint, or generalised poor posture. The two sacroiliac joints are found on either side of the bottom of the spine at the back.
- You have recently been inactive or gained weight.
- You do excessive exercise or have muscle strain.

Before presuming that your pain is muscle or joint pain, it is important to exclude other conditions. Conditions that are easily confused with this pain include a prolapsed vertebral disc, a nerve caught in scar tissue, or medical conditions like fibromyalgia, arthritis, multiple sclerosis or systemic lupus erythematosus (SLE). Your general practitioner can help you exclude these conditions. Fibromyalgia has generalised muscle tenderness rather than isolated tender spots.

What can I do about muscle or joint pelvic pain?

Recognising which factors have caused your pain is a large part of managing the problem. If your pain is due to poor muscle tone from inactivity, then exercises and improving your general health are important. If your pain is due to too much activity with muscle fatigue, then rest and modifying or avoiding the aggravating activity helps. Whatever the cause, you have developed tension and irritability in a group of muscles or a joint.

The best treatment for you will depend on the cause of the problem. A physiotherapist with an interest in pelvic conditions or trigger point therapy is a good person to see for this problem. The treatments that they may recommend include:

- *Specific work on your tender areas.* This includes therapeutic massage, pressure therapies, myofascial release therapy, heat therapy and ultrasound treatment.
- *Exercises* to improve your posture, stretch tight muscles (this decreases trigger point activation) and improve the strength in weak muscles around the joints.
- *Consider your general health.* Low levels of B-group vitamins, low thyroid function and low blood sugar levels can all aggravate muscle irritability.
- *A 'TENS' machine.* This is a small machine the size of a pack of cards. Two small sticky pads are placed over the tender area, and electricity passed between the two pads. This blocks pain impulses going to the brain from that area. It should be set at a

level where you notice a gentle tingling sensation and should not be painful.

- *Cool and stretch technique.* A physiotherapist uses a cooling spray to decrease pain around the tender point, and the muscle is then stretched to its full length. This treatment can be repeated daily, usually for one or two weeks, and should provide rapid results. It is only suitable for muscles on the exterior of the body. If the muscles become sore, the treatment should be stopped for a few days.

- *Needle injection of the tender area with an anaesthetic.* It is actually the needle in the tender point rather than the anaesthetic that helps the pain, but without the anaesthetic, the procedure would be too painful. Needling brings pain relief, but must be repeated weekly for around six weeks. If you don't improve over this time, there may be other factors contributing to your pain.

- *Acupuncture.* Acupuncture has been used to treat pain for centuries. However, it should be seen as an opportunity to manage the pain while you correct the underlying problem, rather than as a complete treatment in itself.

- *Treatment for anxiety or depression.* Both anxiety and depression cause muscular pain by increasing muscle tension. They may not have caused your pain, but they can slow your recovery.

- *Medications.* Some tender areas in muscle are due to irritation at the place where the nerve joins the muscle. There are some features in common with neuropathic pain. Anti-inflammatory medications (see Chapter 6, page 63) and low dose amitriptyline (see page 72) often help muscular pain. Botox will relax overly tense vaginal muscles for up to 6 months.

If treatment is effective and an active tender point settles, then your pain should resolve. However, unless the original cause of the problem is fixed, the tender point, *and the pain* may return. This means that some long-term changes in posture, exercise or general condition are needed. An excellent book for anyone with muscle or joint pain is *Explain Pain* written by D. Butler and G. Moseley (see Reference 22).

Arthritis as a cause of pelvic pain

Sita is a 45-year-old doctor who had developed chronic pelvic pain over two years. She had always had some pain with periods and suspected that she had adenomyosis in her uterus (see page 151). Her pain was worse at period time, but could come at any time of the month.

Sita had a hysterectomy, but was disappointed to find that although her period pain had gone, her other pelvic pain continued. After many tests, Sita was found to have early onset arthritis in her spine with pain 'referred' to her pelvis.

Four different causes of pain

Misha is an 18-year-old university student, referred for removal of endometriosis found at a laparoscopy. On discussion, Misha had four separate causes for her pain! Removing her endometriosis would only treat one of her pains and leave her disappointed. Her four pains were:

- Muscular pain referred to her pelvis. After horse riding, or working with a hoe in local vineyards, her period pain was much more severe. During a few months of study for her exams, where she neither rode horses, nor worked in the vineyard, her period pain improved.
- Bowel pain. At any time of the month, bloating and pelvic pain could occur. After passing a bowel action, her

symptoms improved. A change in diet, investigation of possible food intolerance, and review by a gastroenterologist were advised.

- Prostaglandin pain. This was the pain felt on the first one or two days of her period. The contraceptive pill or an anti-prostaglandin medication would help.
- Endometriosis pain. The endometriosis should be removed.

Who can help me with muscular or joint pain?

- A physiotherapist with an interest in pelvic conditions.
- A pain clinic.
- Your general practitioner if he or she has an interest in this area.
- A sex counsellor if you have tight vaginal muscles.

6 Pain from the bladder — interstitial cystitis

You may know all about cystitis. If so, you probably mean *bacterial cystitis* which is the medical word for a bladder infection. Bacteria get into the bladder, grow there, and irritate the bladder wall. A bladder infection gets better with antibiotics because they kill the bacteria that cause the infection.

The word 'cystitis' really only means an inflammation (irritation) of the bladder. It does not say what caused the inflammation. Interstitial cystitis (IC) is different from bacterial cystitis. There is irritation of the bladder wall but no infection. Antibiotics don't help because there are no bacteria present.

IC is a poorly understood condition. What *is* understood is that it can cause long-term pelvic pain and that it is more common in women with endometriosis. Although some men get interstitial cystitis, it is ten times more common in women.

Even though IC is not a bacterial infection, women with IC often get more bladder infections than other women. Any IC symptoms usually worsen during and after a urine infection.

For reasons that are not well understood, women with IC often *also* have an irritable bowel (see page 160), fibromyalgia (generalised muscle pain), vulvar vestibulitis (a painful area near the opening of the vagina), migraines or allergies as well as their IC. They may also have endometriosis. This makes the pain of IC complicated to both diagnose and manage.

Like endometriosis, many women with IC suffer pain for years before the correct diagnosis is made. This is very distressing. Just like endometriosis, IC is now receiving more attention than before. There have been significant improvements in the way IC is treated, and it is diagnosed much more frequently now than in the past.

What type of pain does interstitial cystitis cause?

The pain may be a burning pain, a shooting pain, a pressure feeling or a spasm. It is felt in the pelvis, in the bladder itself or in the urethra (the tube carrying urine out of the bladder). Commonly, the *pain* worsens as the bladder fills and improves as the bladder empties.

Women with IC usually have other bladder symptoms such as *frequency* (wanting to go to the toilet often), *urgency* (needing to go the toilet in a hurry), and *nocturia* (needing to get up to the toilet at night). Intercourse may be painful, especially in positions that put pressure on the bladder.

The pain may be aggravated by intercourse, periods or foods that are high in acid or potassium. Stress does not cause IC, but it can certainly make it worse.

How is IC diagnosed?

There is no one good test for IC. Really it is what doctors call a 'clinical diagnosis'. This means that if the symptoms fit IC and no other cause for the symptoms is found, then IC is diagnosed. To exclude other causes of pain you may need:

- A urine test to exclude a urine infection or the presence of cancer cells. If there are white cells in the urine but no infection, then you should be checked for Chlamydia infection.
- A bladder diary, which records how much urine you pass, and how often you pass it over a few days.
- An ultrasound of the kidney, pelvic organs and bladder.
- Review by a urologist to check that other conditions are not present, and,
- A short operation called a **cystoscopy** where a telescope is inserted through the urethra into the bladder. A cystoscopy looks at the inside surface of the bladder.

A cystoscopy done in women with IC usually looks normal, but can be useful to exclude other problems such as endometriosis inside the bladder (uncommon) or other causes of bladder irritation such as bladder stones or bladder cancer.

How can I treat my IC?

There are probably several types of IC currently put together in one group, so it is not surprising that no one treatment helps everyone. For some women, dietary changes are enough to manage their symptoms, while others need the experience of a doctor who specialises in bladder and kidney problems (urologist) to work through the treatment options until a suitable option is found. As more becomes known about IC over the next few years, it will become easier to fit the right treatment to the right person.

Usually it is a matter of working through a number of treatments with your doctor until you find one that works for you. No treatment works in everyone and unfortunately no treatment usually works forever. Luckily about 10 per cent of women spontaneously get better over time. The treatment options include:

- *Dietary changes*. Drinks that are high in potassium, acid or caffeine such as fruit juices (including cranberry juice), fizzy drinks, coffee, tea or alcohol should be avoided. The best fluid to drink is water. Diet advice for IC is available at http://www.ichelp.com/TreatmentAndSelfHelp/ICAndDiet.html

- *Drinking the right amount of fluid for you*. This may mean drinking more (to dilute the urine and avoid bladder irritation), or drinking less (if the extra fluid aggravates your symptoms). Around two litres of water a day suits most women.

- *Exercise and stress reduction*. IC is not due to stress, but stress makes it worse. Some women find meditation, hypnosis, massage and relaxation therapies useful. Hot or cold packs placed between the legs, warm baths, wearing loose clothing/belts and cotton underwear may also help.

- *Bladder retraining*. Learning to hold on longer is worthwhile. A continence physiotherapist can show you how to retrain your bladder and improve your pelvic floor.

- *Amitriptyline* (see Chapter 6, page 72). Even low doses help frequency, urgency, pain and voiding at night.

- *Pentosan polysulphate sodium* (Elmiron). This is a tablet of glycosaminoglycan, a substance that protects the inside of the bladder from irritation. The dose is 100 mg three times daily. It helps around 40 per cent of people and may take up to six months to work. Possible side effects include diarrhoea, dyspepsia, reversible hair loss, headache, rash and occasionally liver function abnormalities.

- *Other medications*. These include anti-histamines such as hydroxyzine, H2-antagonists such as cimetidine,

Resiniferotoxin, Botox injections into the bladder wall, anti-spasm medications such as oxybutynin (Ditropan) and muscle relaxants such as tolteradine (Detrusitol).

- *Hydrodistension of the bladder.* The bladder is over-filled with salty water (saline) under a general anaesthetic to stretch its wall. After the bladder has been stretched, 90 per cent of women with IC will show a special pattern of bleeding in the bladder wall. Around 60 per cent of women will have fewer IC symptoms in the months after a hydrodistension.
- *Bladder instillations.* These are medicines mixed with fluid and put inside the bladder. They settle bladder irritation. They include dimethyl sulfoxide (DMSO), bacillus calmette-guerin, Chlorpactin steroids, heparin, local anaesthetics, and hyaluronic acid.
- *Transcutaneous Electrical Nerve Stimulation.* A TENS machine, (sometimes used for pain relief in childbirth) helps some women.
- *Sacral nerve neurostimulators.* These devices stimulate the bladder electrically. They are implanted in the buttock and stimulate nerves to the bladder.
- *Urethral dilatation.* This is rarely used nowadays.
- *Major surgery.* Surgery to remove part of the bladder is *rarely* necessary unless all else has failed.

First aid for a painful bladder

If there are times when your pain or urgency comes on quickly, drink 500ml of water mixed with 1 teaspoon of bicarbonate of soda. Then drink 250ml of water every 20 minutes over the next few hours. If pain persists, try ibuprofen or paracetamol. If no better, have a urine test for infection and only take antibiotics if an infection is found.

Pelvic pain due to interstitial cystitis and endometriosis

Niamh is a 26-year-old whose endometriosis was diagnosed and removed at a laparoscopy four years ago. Her period pain improved, but over time she developed a new type of pain. This pain was above her pubic bone, worse if she delayed passing urine, and better once some urine had been passed. It was also worse after intercourse, whenever she was anxious or after drinking fruit juice, soft drinks or red wine. She passed urine frequently and could not 'hold on' as well as before.

A urine sample showed no sign of infection, but did show tiny amounts of white blood cells. A cystoscopy done by a urologist was normal.

Niamh worked on her diet, stress and the type of drinks she chose. She started a small dose of amitriptyline taken each night (see Chapter 6, page 72).

Six weeks later, her pain was 50 per cent better, but she still passed urine often. Her urologist recommended a small dose of oxybutynin to slow the bladder muscle. This improved her symptoms even more. Niamh still has some pain, but it is now manageable.

Who can help me with bladder pain?

- A urologist.
- A physiotherapist with an interest in pelvic conditions and bladder function.
- Your general practitioner if he or she has an interest in this area.
- A gynaecologist if they have an interest in this area.
- A pain clinic if other treatments have failed.

7 Pain from the ovaries

Anything that stretches or ties down an ovary can cause pain. Ovaries are important and sensitive organs and they don't like it!

What type of pain is ovarian pain?

This depends on whether or not your pelvis is otherwise normal, or you have a pelvic condition aggravating one or both ovaries.

If you have a normal-looking pelvis, you have not reached menopause and you are neither pregnant nor on the contraceptive pill, then normal ovulation pain is common. You may notice a deep ache on one or other side of the lower pelvis lasting from a few hours to a day that happens each month almost exactly 14 days before a period arrives. As the ovaries usually take it in turns to ovulate, normal ovulation pain swaps sides most months. If one of your ovaries has been removed, then the ovary that remains will ovulate each month and the pain will be on the same side each month. Not all women with a normal pelvis get ovulation pain.

If you have a pelvic condition, such as adhesions or endometriosis, affecting an ovary then your pain will last for longer, and be more severe in the months when it is that ovary's turn to ovulate. Anything that ties down the ovary makes ovulation pain worse, because the ovary is not free to change size and shape freely. The pain will still be worst around ovulation time, but may bother you at other times of the month too. If both ovaries are affected, then the ache will affect both sides of your pelvis.

Functional ovarian cysts and ovarian remnant syndrome cause slightly different types of ovarian pain.

What can I do about normal ovulation pain?

- *Do nothing.* Ovulation pain is not dangerous.
- *Take anti-prostaglandin medications* (see Chapter 6, page 63). Prostaglandin chemicals are released at ovulation, so these medications help, especially if they are taken before the pain is too severe.
- *Use a contraceptive pill.* Most Pills stop ovulation, but some of the newer very low dose Pills do not.
- *Use a progestogen only contraceptive* such as Implanon.

Functional ovarian cysts

Functional cysts are cysts that form as part of the function of the ovary. It is normal for an ovary to make small, round, fluid-filled cysts from time to time in women who are neither pregnant nor on the contraceptive Pill. Most are not painful, but some are.

If they do cause pain, it is a constant ache, felt most of the time on one side of the pelvis. It may last a few weeks or a few months, but ultimately goes away by itself. As functional cysts can make hormones, periods become irregular and some women notice tender breasts. If the cyst pops (ruptures), there is a sudden pain that goes away a few hours later. Functional cysts don't cause long-term pain so they are rarely confused with endometriosis.

Importantly, there is another condition that can cause a sudden pain in one side of the lower pelvis, irregular periods and breast tenderness: *an ectopic pregnancy.* An ectopic pregnancy is a pregnancy in the fallopian tube rather than in the uterus. It is a dangerous condition and easy to confuse with a functional cyst. If you are unsure, see your doctor. A good quality pregnancy test will be positive in women with an ectopic pregnancy and negative in women with a functional cyst.

How can I know if I have a functional cyst?

- An ultrasound scan shows a cyst that looks like a round balloon filled with clear watery fluid. It should be less than 5 cm across and have no solid pieces inside it. If it has ruptured, then the ultrasound may be normal or show a small amount of fluid in your pelvis, and
- *Your pregnancy test is negative.*

What can I do about functional cysts?

- *Do nothing.* Most functional cysts go away within two or three months. You may wish to have another ultrasound scan two or three months later to ensure that it has resolved.
- *Start the contraceptive pill.* This may not remove your cyst, but will help prevent more functional cysts in the future.
- *A laparoscopy with removal of the cyst.* This is only necessary if your doctor is unsure what type of cyst it is, or your pain cannot be managed. Even if the cyst is removed, this does not prevent other cysts forming.

Ovarian remnant syndrome

This syndrome describes pain or a pelvic mass in a woman who has had both her ovaries (and often her uterus) removed in the past. A small piece of ovary has been left behind *unintentionally* at her operation, and has enlarged and become painful. It usually occurs in women who have had a lot of pelvic surgery in the past and had many adhesions in their pelvis. The gynaecologist who did their operation did not intend to leave behind any ovary at all, but scar tissue or endometriosis made removing the ovary difficult. Over time, even a tiny piece of ovary can respond to hormonal signals from the brain and grow or make cysts.

What type of pain does it cause?

Ovarian remnants cause pain that is felt on one side of the pelvis. In younger women, the pain is worst about once a month, when ovulation would have been, but in older women it can cause chronic pain. Not all ovarian remnants cause pain, but those that do, start to cause problems within a few years of surgery.

How is it diagnosed?

Your description of the pain is the most useful way to diagnose an ovarian remnant. Other ways include:

*   *A blood test for oestrogen or FSH.* If you have had both ovaries removed, and are not using HRT then you should have low levels of oestrogen and high levels of FSH (a hormone made by the brain). If your oestrogen levels are normal or your FSH is low then it is likely that a small piece of active ovary remains.
*   *An ultrasound scan* may show a cyst in the pelvis that has formed in the remaining piece of ovary.
*   *A laparoscopy.* The ovarian remnant looks like white, often cystic, scar tissue. Sometimes a medication called clomiphene citrate is used before surgery to make the remnant larger and easier to find.

What can I do about an ovarian remnant?

Any treatment that removes the ovarian remnant or makes it less active will help the pain. These options include:

*   *No treatment.* At menopause the remnant will become less active, just as a normal ovary does, and your pain *might* improve.
*   *Medications to make the ovarian remnant less active.* The Pill, a GnRH analogue (see Chapter 6, page 67) or a continuous progestogen medication (see Chapter 6, page 75) usually help.

- *An operation to remove the ovarian remnant.* This surgery can be difficult because most remnants are small and trapped among scar tissue. They lie close to the ureter, which is easily damaged during surgery. The good thing about removing the remnant is that the pain usually resolves.
- *Radiotherapy.* The same radiation treatment used to treat some cancers can be used to make the ovary inactive. This is an uncommon treatment nowadays.

Who can help me with ovarian pain?

- Your general practitioner (for ovulation pain or functional cysts).
- Your normal gynaecologist (for ovulation pain or functional cysts).
- A laparoscopic surgeon (gynaecologist) for removal of an ovarian remnant.

8 Pain from veins – ovarian vein syndrome and pelvic congestion syndrome

Just as some enlarged (varicose) veins in the legs ache, varicose veins in the pelvis can ache too. If it is the ovarian vein that is enlarged, then the condition is called ovarian vein syndrome (OVS), whereas if it is the veins around the uterus that are enlarged, it is called pelvic congestion syndrome (PCS). Both conditions are commonest in women who have had children and are aged in their twenties and thirties.

What type of pain can veins cause?

The commonest pain is a generalised dull ache felt in one or both sides of the pelvis. It is worse after standing for long periods of time, straining to pass a bowel action or walking, because these activities encourage congestion in the pelvic veins. Sometimes just changing position is enough to bring on the pain.

As a period comes closer, the pelvis becomes even more congested, the pain worsens and a painful period follows. Painful intercourse on deep penetration is very common, as is an ache after intercourse. Other symptoms include a low backache and, in some women, occasional sharp pains.

Lying down reduces the pelvic congestion and improves the pain, just as it does for varicose leg veins, so most women with pelvic congestion still sleep well.

Why does it happen?

In the past, pelvic congestion syndrome was thought to be more common in women who found orgasm difficult. Nowadays, few doctors believe this theory. Changes in the way veins carry blood are a more likely cause.

Veins are thin-walled blood vessels that carry blood back from the pelvis to the heart. To help them do this, they have valves that allow blood to move forwards but not backwards. This helps the blood travel upwards when you stand up. If the valves don't work, the blood does not return to the heart as efficiently and it collects in the veins of the pelvis. The pressure from this blood causes congestion in the pelvic organs and stretches the wall of the vein. The vein becomes enlarged and 'varicose'.

How are varicose pelvic veins diagnosed?

- *Examination* of the labia, thigh or buttocks *may* show enlarged veins in these areas too.
- *A doppler ultrasound scan* shows an enlarged vein and poor vein valve function. The left ovarian vein is affected much more commonly than the right.
- *A venogram* is an X-ray test that shows the size and position of

the veins in the pelvis. A dye is injected into the pelvis and an X-ray picture taken. Where doppler ultrasound is available, a venogram is rarely necessary.

- *A laparoscopy* may show enlarged veins in the pelvis.

Just having enlarged pelvic veins does not mean that they are the cause for your pain. An Israeli study (see Reference 23) looked at women with pelvic pain and an enlarged left ovarian vein, who were already booked for surgery to donate one of their kidneys. During this operation it is usual to divide the ovarian vein. It was a good opportunity to see if dividing the vein also helped their pelvic pain. After the operation, half the women were better, but half were not. This suggests that some of them had pain due to their enlarged ovarian vein, but for others their pain had another cause.

What can I do about enlarged ovarian or pelvic veins?

The best treatment for you will depend on which veins are varicose and whether these veins are truly the cause of your pelvic pain.

- *No treatment.* Unless your pain is severe, this may be your best option. The enlarged veins may not be the cause of your pain.
- *Treat other health problems.* By treating other conditions such as heavy periods (see Chapter 9, page 158), emotional distress (see Chapter 11, page 219), and premenstrual tension, you may find your pelvic pain improves or becomes easier to live with.
- *Surgery to divide (ligate) an enlarged ovarian vein.* The best operation depends on which veins are enlarged and whether or not you have completed your family. If it is the ovarian vein that is enlarged, it can be divided by removing the ovary on that side, or by dividing the vein and leaving the ovary. Dividing the vein and leaving the ovary is a much more difficult operation.

- *Surgery to ligate enlarged pelvic veins.* This involves removing the uterus (a hysterectomy). An operation to divide the veins and leave the uterus is currently impractical. A hysterectomy will also treat pain from the uterus itself, and heavy periods.
- *Embolisation of the enlarged vein.* An X-ray doctor (radiologist) inserts a small tube through a blood vessel in your groin and passes it through to the enlarged vein. A substance is injected into the vein to block (embolise) it.

Even women who choose a hysterectomy with both ovaries removed do not always find that their pain goes completely. There are many unanswered questions about pelvic congestion syndrome and the best way to manage the pain it causes. All these procedures have risks, so you should discuss them carefully with your doctor. He or she will know what services are available in your area, and what they would recommend for your individual situation.

Who can help me with vein pain?

- Your gynaecologist, particularly if they are skilled at laparoscopic surgery. It requires laparoscopic skills to exclude other conditions such as endometriosis, remove an ovary through the laparoscope, divide the ovarian vein and remove the uterus through small cuts if you choose a hysterectomy.
- A radiologist working with your gynaecologist.

9 Pain from the appendix

If you have had *appendicitis* you will know that you became sick quite quickly, over a few days. You had a high temperature, pain on the right side of your lower abdomen, looked sick to those around you, and then had an operation to remove your appendix. This is the common way in which an appendix causes pain.

But can the appendix cause long-term pain without ever

developing actual appendicitis? This is something that doctors disagree on. Some believe it can, but most believe that unless the appendix is infected, it does not cause pain.

A recently reported American study (see Reference 24) studied 300 women who had chronic pain on the right side, no abnormality found at a laparoscopy and a normal-looking appendix removed. Of these women 10 per cent found that their pain had gone after their surgery. This, of course, also means that 90 per cent of these women were no better.

Would their pain have gone away even without surgery, or did removing the normal-looking appendix actually help them? It is difficult to know.

Certainly if the appendix is affected by abnormalities that can be seen, such as endometriosis, then it is best removed.

What pain might the appendix cause?

It might cause pain in the lower right side of the abdomen.

What is the appendix?

The appendix is part of the bowel. It is a hollow tube, closed at one end and opening into an important part of the bowel called the *caecum* at the other end. The appendix is about the same shape and size as a woman's little finger. If it becomes blocked and infected with bacteria this causes *appendicitis*. An operation to remove it is called an *appendicectomy* or an *appendectomy*. Acute appendicitis is not a cause of long-term pain.

What treatment is available for appendix pain?

As no useful role for the appendix has been found in humans, if it causes problems, then it is removed. This can almost always be done through a laparoscope.

Treating actual appendicitis, or removing an appendix that lies in a difficult position requires a bowel surgeon, but in other situations a gynaecologist skilled in laparoscopic surgery may be able to remove it for you.

Removing the appendix usually goes smoothly, but complications are possible, and many gynaecologists are not trained in this type of surgery. For this reason, it is only done in women who have symptoms that could fit with appendix pain, or in women where abnormalities of the appendix (such as endometriosis) are seen at their surgery.

Who can help me with appendix pain?

- A laparoscopic surgeon (gynaecologist) as part of your endometriosis surgery.
- A laparoscopic surgeon (bowel surgeon).

10 Endosalpingiosis (serous change)

Sometimes a white lesion that was thought to be endometriosis is found to be endosalpingiosis when checked by a pathologist. So what is the difference between endometriosis and endo-salpingiosis?

End*ometriosis is tissue that looks a little like the lining of the uterus.*

End*osalpingiosis is tissue that looks a little like the lining of the fallopian tube.*

The two conditions are similar but certainly not the same. Just like endometriosis, it can only be diagnosed with a laparoscopy. It may look just the same as endometriosis, but once it is sent to a pathologist, they can pick the difference when they look at it through a microscope.

Doctors disagree as to whether or not endosalpingiosis causes pain.

A German study looked at over 1000 women having a laparoscopy during one year. They found endosalpingiosis in 7 per cent of these women. It was just as common in women with pelvic pain, as in women without pelvic pain (see Reference 25).

However, many laparoscopic surgeons have treated women whose pain has improved after removal of endosalpingiosis. It may be that tiny areas of endosalpingiosis are normal and painless, while larger areas might be painful. There is more to learn about this condition.

Who can help me with endosalpingiosis?

- A laparoscopic surgeon (gynaecologist). These operations require the same skill as endometriosis surgery.

11 Pelvic infection (pelvic inflammatory disease)

It is normal for a woman to have bacteria in the vagina and cervix, but not in the uterus, fallopian tubes, around the ovaries or in the abdominal cavity. A pelvic infection means that these areas have become infected. The infection may be *acute*, which means that it came on quickly and has only been present for a short time, or *chronic* which means that it has been present for some time. Some women have repeated acute infections, never completely recovering between bouts of infection.

There may be a mixture of bacteria present. Some, such as gonorrhoea or chlamydia, are transmitted sexually while others are just the normal bacteria living in our bowel or vagina all the time.

What type of pain do pelvic infections cause?

An acute infection can cause a wide variety of symptoms. Some women become very sick quite rapidly. They have a high temperature, severe pain across both sides of their lower abdomen and may vomit. They look sick. There may be an increase in the vaginal discharge or abnormal vaginal bleeding. Other women have mild pelvic pain, but nothing severe enough to cause them to see a doctor. This type of infection can easily go unrecognised.

Over time, infection can damage the fallopian tubes and cause adhesions. If the fallopian tubes become blocked, they fill with fluid and enlarge. This is called a *hydrosalpinx*. Infection and adhesions around the fallopian tube and ovary on one side may form a tender mass called an abscess. These long-term problems can cause chronic pelvic pain.

Some women only find out that they have had a pelvic infection in the past when they have a laparoscopy to investigate why they have not become pregnant easily. The infection had blocked their fallopian tubes.

Occasionally, there is pain and tenderness over the liver in the upper right segment of the abdomen. This is due to adhesions around the liver and has a special name (Fitz-Hugh-Curtis syndrome).

Can pelvic infections be prevented?

Safer sexual practices including the use of barrier contraception (condoms and diaphragms) decrease the risk of catching the sexually transmitted infections that commonly cause pelvic infections.

Vaginal douching should be avoided.

How is a pelvic infection diagnosed?

- *A doctor's examination* of the pelvis may show tender areas on both sides of the lower abdomen, an increased vaginal discharge, and tenderness on vaginal examination when the cervix is moved from side to side. Occasionally a hydrosalpinx or abscess near the ovary is found.
- *Swabs* taken from the cervix may show infection with chlamydia or gonorrhoea. Nowadays, a urine specimen can

check for chlamydia infection too. To do this, the laboratory needs the first few drops of urine you pass in the morning, rather than the 'mid-stream' urine specimen that checks for a bladder infection. If you are told that a sexual partner of yours has chlamydia, you need to be checked for infection too.

- *Blood tests* for white blood cells, C-reactive protein and ESR may show high values. These tests look for infection or inflammation anywhere in the body.
- *An ultrasound* may be normal, but may show a dilated tube, ovarian cyst or ovarian abscess.
- *A laparoscopy.* This is the most reliable test. It shows red inflamed pelvic organs and sometimes pus, as well as a hydrosalpinx or abscess if they are present.

A laparoscopy is not always necessary but if there is any doubt about whether or not you have a pelvic infection, it can be very useful. Without a laparoscopy, many women have their pain labelled as PID, which may or may not be true. From then on any pain they have may be considered as just another infection.

While a laparoscopy is useful to *diagnose* a pelvic infection, it is best to leave any major surgery until the pelvic infection has been treated. If surgery is done during an infection, there is a high chance that severe pelvic adhesions may form.

How is a pelvic infection treated?

A pelvic infection is treated with antibiotics. Which antibiotics are used will depend on how sick you are, what type of bacteria you have, and whether or not you have been admitted to hospital. Most women have more than one type of bacteria causing their infection, so they need more than one antibiotic. You may be prescribed:

- One antibiotic for a group of bacteria that include chlamydia (as well as similar bacteria that are not sexually transmitted)
- One antibiotic for a group of bacteria called 'anaerobes', and

- One antibiotic for other bacteria.

Your partner may need antibiotics too. If so, it is important that you both take the antibiotics at the same time, to avoid re-infecting each other

If you are very sick, you may be admitted to hospital so that your antibiotics can be given to you through an intravenous (IV) drip. Whatever you need, it is important that your infection be treated. The longer it is there, the more damage it can do, and the more likely it is that your pain could become chronic.

Who can help me with a pelvic infection?

- Your general practitioner.
- A gynaecologist.

12 Pelvic Inflammation (without infection)

Sometimes tissue that looks like endometriosis at a laparoscopy, is found to be 'inflamed tissue' when it is removed and checked with a microscope. Recent research suggests that this might be an 'autoimmune' condition (See Ref 28). Autoimmune conditions are those where the body makes antibodies to itself, which can damage normal tissues.

What sort of pain does it cause?

This varies but most women have sharp stabbing pain, worse before periods. Tiredness, pain with sex and extra-sensitive skin are common.

How is it diagnosed?

- Biopsy at laparoscopy shows chronic (long term) inflammation

- Blood tests for the immune system. The C-Reactive Protein, Erythrocyte Sedimentation Rate and blood picture are often abnormal
- Blood tests for auto-immune antibodies such as anti-nuclear antibodies, thyroid antibodies, rheumatoid factor etc.

How can it be treated?

- Excising the area at laparoscopy may be enough
- Anti-inflammatory medications (See page 63)
- Auto-immune medications. These are medications more commonly used for rheumatoid arthritis, or SLE such as hydroxychloroquine (200 mg twice daily) or methotrexate (up to 10 mg weekly).

Who can help me with my pain?

Few doctors associate auto-immune conditions with pelvic pain. You could discuss Reference 28 with your doctor.

Chapter 10

. . . .

You and your gynaecologist

I F YOU FEEL NERVOUS at the thought of seeing a gynaecologist, you are not alone. Most people do. Not only does your visit concern a private part of your body, but also the outcome of your visit is important to you. If it goes well, you may be on the path to less pain.

How to choose a gynaecologist

Obstetrics and gynaecology cover a large field: too large for all gynaecologists to be expert in all areas. We all specialise to some degree. Some doctors specialise in laparoscopic surgery and endometriosis.

Your general practitioner (GP) knows the services available in your area, and if you have a choice will try to refer you to a gynaecologist who suits your personality and needs. If you will be attending a public hospital, ask which hospital has a good reputation for laparoscopic surgery. This increases the likelihood that the doctor you see will have a good understanding of endometriosis. There is very little endometriosis surgery that cannot be done through a laparoscope, but these skills are not available everywhere.

What is an Obstetrician and Gynaecologist?

An obstetrician cares for women when they are pregnant.

A gynaecologist cares for women when they are not pregnant.

To become an Obstetrician and Gynaecologist (often called an 'O and G' or ObGyn) requires a minimum of a medical degree followed by specialist training over several years in this area. After completing specialist training, some O and Gs specialise further in a particular area of gynaecology, while others continue to work in both areas. So a gynaecologist is also an obstetrician, but may or may not still deliver babies.

Endometriosis surgery is difficult surgery. There are great benefits to be had, but there are also risks. No surgeon seeks to hurt their patients and no surgeon likes complications. It is important to us that our patients are happy with the care we provide. Because of this some gynaecologists choose *not* to do endometriosis surgery because it is not their area of expertise. This is a very reasonable and responsible choice.

All gynaecologists spend time each year in training. In some countries this is compulsory if we wish to continue working as gynaecologists. However, there are many areas of training we can choose, so we all develop different areas of interest. Most gynaecologists are able to diagnose endometriosis by laparoscopy, but only some are able to do the more complicated surgery necessary to remove the endometriosis completely.

Learning and maintaining the skills necessary for modern

endometriosis surgery is a heavy commitment for a gynaecologist. It requires time away from work, and significant expense. Operating close to delicate organs on a regular basis also adds that extra stress to a surgeon's life that some doctors wisely decide they do not need. If your current gynaecologist has areas of expertise outside endometriosis he or she may refer you to another gynaecologist, especially if your endometriosis is severe. If, after reading Chapter 9, your pain may be due to something else apart from endometriosis, then you should see one of the professionals recommended in that section rather than your endometriosis surgeon.

If the gynaecologist you are considering is a friend or relative of yours, you may be better to consider a different doctor. Your doctor friend will want everything to go smoothly for you; yet can provide no more guarantee of this than for any other patient. It is very difficult to be both doctor and friend, and your non-medical relationship may suffer. In some circumstances there may be no other suitable alternative, but if there is a choice, you can always ask him or her whom they would recommend.

Finally, it is important that you feel some rapport with your doctor. If problems occur, a good relationship will help both you and your doctor through a difficult time. If you don't feel comfortable with your gynaecologist, ask your GP or gynaecologist for a second opinion. Your doctor will not be offended. We all have patients with whom a useful relationship develops easily, and others with whom it is more difficult.

You should also ask for a second opinion if you believe that your pain is not being taken seriously.

> It is sometimes said that there is a doctor for every patient and a patient for every doctor, but no doctor who suits everyone.

I have had pain for SO long and I am SO angry

You may have a lot of reasons to be angry. Severe pain, disappointments, having your pain ignored or being treated badly is enough to make anyone angry. You may be angry because a treatment failed, and life seems unfair, even when you know that those who cared for you did their best. Anger can be a positive thing if it helps you keep going, but it is not helpful if it prevents you moving forward to recovery.

A new doctor is a new opportunity to look at your pain afresh. Difficult though it is, it is important to give a new doctor the opportunity to do *their* best. To you, he or she may be just another doctor. To them, you are a new person and a new challenge.

Some women only feel able to express anger to those doctors who listen most and treat them well. They feel unable to tell those they dislike how they feel. It is important that you are able to explain how you feel about past treatments, but where anger runs deep it can interfere with your new professional relationship. More importantly, it can interfere with your care and treatment. This is not in your interest.

If you feel unable to move forward due to fear, disappointment or anger, then this needs to be resolved. A counsellor may be the best person to talk to about your feelings. He or she is someone who is not part of your medical care, not a member of your family and not a friend. You can talk freely.

Preparation for your visit, and what to ask

Your first visit to the gynaecologist is a first for both of you. He or she does not know the type of person you are, nor what you are looking for. Time must be spent talking about your pain, any previous treatments, and going through the options you have now.

I find that two women with exactly the same symptoms may make completely different treatment choices. Some wish to avoid surgery at all costs, even if that means living with pain, whereas others think of surgery as their first choice.

Something as complicated as pelvic pain takes time to work through. If you are well prepared for your visit, then less time is spent going through the basic information your doctor needs, and more time can be spent learning about your condition, and considering which options would suit *you* best. After all, the most important thing to come away with is a plan with which you are happy.

Being prepared for your visit means thinking about the questions you may be asked beforehand. In my practice we ask women to fill in a short questionnaire at home before their appointment. This allows them time to think about the answers and look up any information if necessary. If all the things they wish to discuss are written down, then they are unlikely to be forgotten on the day. Your gynaecologist will appreciate the care you have taken.

The questions a gynaecologist usually asks might concern:

- *Your periods.* Are they regular? How long is it between the first day of one period and the first day of the next period (cycle length)? Are they heavy or light? Are they painful? Do you have bleeding between your periods?
- *Your pain.* When do you get pain? Is it related to periods, and if so, during which days? What makes it better? What makes it worse? Does it wake you at night? Where is it? Does the pain move to any other areas?
- *Your bladder and bowel function.* Are these normal? Do they cause pain? If so, do you think the bladder or bowel pain is related to your periods?
- *Your sexual relationship, if relevant.* Does intercourse hurt? If so, where do you think the pain is? What contraception are you

using? Are there any other sexual problems you wish to discuss?

- *Treatments you have tried.* Do any medications help your pain? Have you had any surgery in the past? If so, when was this, what was found, what was done, and did it help?

- *Any plans for pregnancy, if relevant.* Are you currently trying to get pregnant? Do you plan a pregnancy in the near future? Have you had a problem becoming pregnant in the past?

- *Your medical history.* Do you have any illnesses? Have you had any other surgery? Were there any problems with anaesthetics? Do you have any allergies?

- *Your family history.* Does anyone else in your family have endometriosis? Is there a history of gynaecological conditions, bleeding disorders, blood clots or drug allergies?

What is a 'normal' period?

Although periods vary widely between different women, they are remarkably similar for each person. Women with *regular* monthly periods usually know how many days they will bleed, how many pads or tampons they will need and when the next period will be. They notice when something is different.

Normal regular periods last between one and eight days (usually five days), occur every 24 to 35 days (usually 28 days), and lose less than 80 ml of blood (usually 50 ml). Whatever cycle length you have, it should be the same, or almost the same each month. If not, then you have irregular periods. Irregular periods are much less predictable. The time between periods varies, periods may be long or short, and the amount of blood lost varies widely.

A period is considered 'heavy' if it is common to pass clots of blood, have 'flooding' or 'accidents' on sheets or clothing, or change pads during the night.

It is not normal to bleed between periods, although sometimes a tiny amount of blood passed only at ovulation time may be normal for you. Bleeding between periods should be reported to your doctor.

Your gynaecologist will be especially pleased to see details of any pelvic operations you have had in the past. This information might include photos from your surgery, an operation sheet describing what was done, or a copy of the letter sent to your general practitioner. The more information your gynaecologist has about your previous surgery, the better they can advise you on future treatment.

It is easy to forget to ask the questions you want answered during your visit. It is best to write your questions down before you go, and check your list before you leave. I do this myself whenever I see a doctor.

If a laparoscopy is planned, ask what type of surgery would be done if endometriosis is found. If your doctor can only offer cautery or laser ablation, then that narrows your options if you are found have endometriosis. These treatments suit some endometriosis, but not all. If you don't feel you have enough information, ask more questions. Frequently, there are different types of surgery possible according to your wishes and individual needs. Be sure that your doctor understands what surgery you want in different situations. They will not be able to ask you while you are asleep.

No-one remembers all that is said during one appointment, especially if they are anxious or in pain. Taking your partner, parent or friend with you is a good idea. Your special person may remember things you missed, and it is good to have someone who heard the same advice you did to talk to later on. You could ask your doctor to list the options you have on a piece of paper to take with you and consider later on.

If, after you leave, you cannot decide what to do, you may need more information or just some time to think about it. You could look at the websites listed in the appendix on page 277, talk to your general practitioner, talk with your family, or make another appointment with your gynaecologist to discuss it further.

> **In the end, there is always the option of 'do nothing' and live with it. Remember that it is your pelvis, and your choice. It is also your responsibility to accept the consequences of the choices that you make.**

Vaginal examinations

No-one enjoys vaginal examinations. This is the time when women say to me: 'Why in the world did you become a gynaecologist?' From a gynaecologist's viewpoint, a vaginal examination is just a way of obtaining information you can't get from questions alone. I appreciate that this is not the way that most women see it!

Embarrassment, although very understandable and probably unavoidable, is unnecessary. As gynaecologists, we examine women every day. Whatever your body shape, tattoo preference or body piercing, it is the person underneath who matters, and with whom we have a professional relationship. Your doctor will not think less of you after a vaginal examination.

> ### I am a virgin. Will the gynaecologist want to examine me?
>
> Probably not, but your doctor may not realise that you are a virgin unless you tell him or her.
>
> Cervical smear tests are not necessary in women until they have been sexually active for at least 12 months. As a virgin you

will not be pregnant, and a sexually transmitted disease is unlikely. So if you have never had intercourse there is less need for your doctor to examine you vaginally. He or she may still wish to check your abdomen, because this shows where your pain is. Your parent or support person can stay with you during the examination if you wish. However, if there is private information you wish to tell the doctor, this is a good opportunity to speak to them alone. An ultrasound can show whether or not your uterus or ovaries are enlarged. If your gynaecologist feels that a vaginal examination *is* important, they can discuss this with you, and explain what will be done.

If you have your period at the time of your appointment, you may choose to re-schedule it to another day. However, your gynaecologist is used to the sight of blood and provided that you are comfortable, will be happy to see you for most conditions regardless. Generally they have spare sanitary pads or tampons if needed, and an examination during a period does help in isolating exactly where the period pain is coming from. Some tests, such as cervical smear tests are not reliable when done during a period, so if you are unsure it is best to ring and ask if your appointment should be changed.

There are two parts to a vaginal examination. The first part is called a *speculum examination*. It involves inserting a vaginal speculum into the vagina so that the cervix and the walls of the vagina can be seen. A vaginal **speculum** is an instrument that holds the vagina open. It is used if you are due for a smear test, if you may have endometriosis of the upper vagina, or to look for other gynaecological problems.

The second part is called a *bimanual examination* because both hands are used. Two fingers of one hand are inserted into the vagina and the other hand is placed on the lower abdomen. A bimanual examination allows your doctor to check the size, tenderness and position of the uterus and ovaries. It is more difficult in larger women. Sometimes lumps (nodules) of endometriosis can be felt along the uterosacral ligaments at the top of the vagina, or in the area between vagina and bowel. You should tell your doctor which parts of your pelvis are tender as this may be where your endometriosis lies.

Vaginal examinations may be especially traumatic for women with a painful pelvis, or those who have been sexually assaulted in the past. If you are anxious about being examined, you should tell your doctor. He or she may be unaware of your feelings and there may be another alternative. No doctor wants to cause pain or emotional distress.

Yes, it is possible.

Amber is a 32-year-old woman who had suffered 17 years of severe chronic pelvic pain. Most nights she was woken by agonising, nauseating pain in her back and pelvis. She had given up on men, sex and smear tests. Any attempt at vaginal examination caused excruciating pain. Her vaginal muscles were overly tense and she had vaginismus (see Chapter 2, page 19). Amber had pain in her pelvis after passing urine, bladder frequency and painful bowel actions at period time. A laparoscopy done a few years before had found 'no endometriosis'.

When we met, she was using very high doses of depo-provera as well as the contraceptive pill to stop her periods altogether. Even so, she had severe pelvic pain day and night. Amber was very courageous, but pain for so long had made her wonder if life was worth living. There were so many aspects to Amber's pain that no single treatment would be enough.

We worked though several treatments:

- 10 mg of amitriptyline at night helped her neuropathic and bladder pain. She could now sleep at night without disturbance.
- A laparoscopy showed that she did indeed have endometriosis, but it had an unusual appearance that is commonly missed. Her back pain improved substantially.
- Amber stopped her depo-provera and contraceptive pill. She did not need contraception, they had not helped her pain and her mood was better without them.
- A Mirena IUD was inserted to treat pain from her uterus and take over from the depo-provera when it wore off and her periods returned.
- Amber realised herself that fizzy drinks and coffee aggravated her bladder pain so she cut them out.
- Review by a urologist and starting ditropan improved her bladder pain even further.
- Counselling for the emotional distress she suffered over many years continued.
- A sex therapist continues to work through the vaginismus with her.

Amber still has some pain, but in her own words she 'has her life back' and the pain is '95 per cent gone'. This process has taken four months to achieve. She is not ready for a relationship yet, but who knows?

Chapter 11

....

Coping with endometriosis

Jane Marsh, RN

EVEN THOUGH ALL THE WOMEN I see have endometriosis, their needs vary. Some women have few problems. Their endometriosis can be treated easily, their general health is good and they feel positive about their life. Other women have had a difficult time with endometriosis over many years. They may have other health problems, or personal issues that seem overwhelming.

We discuss practical ways to cope with the effects of endometriosis on their day-to-day lives. Like all of us, women with endometriosis have stresses in their lives that are nothing to do with their disease. We look at practical ways they can help themselves.

This chapter includes a few of the common situations women with endometriosis talk to me about. It provides ideas for working through them. It is divided into ways you can support yourself and ways in which others can support you. Luckily, very few women have all these problems!

Supporting yourself

Coping better with the pain

Pain is a very personal thing. No two women have the same pain and no-one else can experience *your* pain as *you* do. Your doctor can explain medical ways to manage and sometimes cure your pain, but the changes you can make yourself are important too. Even when your medical treatment has been successful, you may still have some pain. Looking after your general health and emotional wellbeing can help you cope better with whatever pain remains.

- *Learn more about your pain.* For some women, finally knowing what it is that has caused them pain for so long, and learning what endometriosis is, helps a lot. The worry that went with an unknown pain is gone, even if the pain itself is still there. Even a laparoscopy that finds no endometriosis can be reassuring. Yes, the need to investigate the pain remains (see Chapter 9) but it is good to know that the pelvis looks healthy. If there are things about your care, or your pain, that you don't under-stand, ask lots of questions.
- *Prioritise your life.* You may find that you can't do *everything* you want to do, so decide what is actually important and what is not.
  - Leave household chores undone if you are not well. At these times, you need to *rest* and look after yourself. You needn't feel guilty – any dust will wait!
  - Avoid taking on more projects or social plans than you can comfortably handle. Pick the important ones and say 'No thank you' to the rest.
  - Make health and being happy together a priority for your family. Your family will function best if you are *all* well, so your needs are important too.

- Where you can, avoid those activities that upset or stress you.

- *Make time for exercise that you* can *do, despite the pain.* Exercise releases chemicals called endorphins that decrease pain. It also distracts your mind from the pain, improves strength, helps with weight loss and makes you feel well. There may be days when you are not well enough to exercise, but do what you can when you can. You can start with gentle exercise, and do more as your strength and endurance improves. Walking, swimming and aquarobics are good exercises to start with.

- *Avoid negative thoughts.* You may have difficult memories of a friend or relative who had serious gynaecological problems. You are an individual and your experience needn't be the same as theirs.

- *Avoid becoming tired.* Your pain will feel worse if you are tired and worn out.
    - Get plenty of sleep.
    - Eat a well-balanced healthy diet to ensure a good intake of vitamins and minerals (see Chapter 12). Avoid alcohol and caffeine. You don't need any 'morning after' feelings.
    - Drink plenty of water. Around 2 litres of fluid daily, is a good goal. Dehydration makes you tired.
    - Encourage and allow your children and partner to do jobs around the house. You don't have to do everything yourself and it will help your children learn to be capable, independent adults.
    - Realise that you needn't be responsible for sorting out every emotional need or disagreement in your family, particularly if they do not involve you directly. There may be things that your family can sort out for themselves.
    - Look for an easier way of doing things. Your partner or children will still love you if they have bought biscuits

rather than home-made ones in their lunchbox. Maybe it's time for them to make their lunch themselves, particularly if you work too.

- *Consider complementary therapies.* An experienced and well-trained therapist might help you. Most of these therapies need persistence and may only work for you while you use them. They are not intended as a replacement for the medications or surgery that your doctor recommends. They can work together with conventional treatments to give you the best result possible.
    - Acupuncture. Acupuncture uses fine needles inserted in the skin at specially chosen places to provide pain relief.
    - Hypnotherapy can help by improving relaxation; making you less aware of your pain and helping you feel more positive about yourself.
    - Herbal and dietary therapies are discussed by Dr Margaret Taylor in Chapter 12.
- When the pain is bad:
    - Use hot packs on your abdomen for warmth and comfort.
    - Take a hot restful bath.
    - If you have children, use what childcare you can afford so that you give yourself a rest. You will be much better company for your children once you feel better.
    - Spend the evening after work in bed. You will be more tired after a day working with pain and you need rest. Your children can come to you to have a book read, or talk about their day. They might really enjoy this time with a more rested and available mother.
    - If you are able to, do something interesting that takes your mind off the pain.

To gain control of your pain you may need to be proactive in seeking out the best treatment available. You may need to mix natural and conventional treatments with a change in your diet, exercise and lifestyle. These are things over which you *do* have control. Remember, your doctor will not be able to fix everything for you. There will be things that you have to do yourself. Working on your health to benefit your pain can benefit your life in other ways too.

Feeling different to your teenage friends

You may think that you are the only teenager ever to have endometriosis, but you are not. It is actually quite common among teenagers. However, if none of the girls you know have it, it is easy to feel 'different' or isolated. Over the years, you may not have understood why your pain was so bad, or why regular period pain medication didn't work for you. Your teachers, friends and parents may not have understood either. They may not have been as supportive as they could have been.

Your local endometriosis support organisation can help you get in touch with other girls your age who also have endometriosis. It is very comforting to talk to girls with a similar experience. It is your choice who you tell about your endometriosis, but you need not feel alone.

Teenagers in general find their relationships at home stressful. Is there someone you trust to whom you can explain what irritates or upsets you? Is there something in particular that worries you? You may have been prescribed the contraceptive pill, yet worry about what this might mean for weight gain, your long-term health or your reputation among your friends.

At your age you have exams and other school expectations to cope with, a growing sexual awareness, skin problems, body image issues, family conflicts and a lot more.

Maintaining your relationships

Endometriosis can strain any relationship: mothers, fathers, siblings, partners, children, workmates, or friends. To avoid this, it is worthwhile explaining to the people that are important to you what endometriosis is and how it affects you. They may have absolutely no understanding of endometriosis, so it is in your best interest to educate them. They won't want to talk about it all the time, but there are some things it is important that they understand.

You should also remember that some of the people in your life may have their own issues to work through once you are diagnosed with endometriosis.

- *Your parents.* It is a parent's natural response to shield their children from any harm or pain. When they can't do this, they may feel guilty, anxious or angry. They may also be scared for you, yet not wish to show it.
- *Your partner.* Your partner may want to 'fix' any problems you have for you, to save you from worry. If they are unable to do so, they may feel useless and unimportant. Tell your partner that you do not expect him (or her) to fix your endometriosis for you, but that you still need their support. There is nothing to see from the outside in a woman with endometriosis, so your pain may be difficult for a man to relate to. They will never have endometriosis themselves and may not understand the pain you are in. Don't presume they understand your pain, or how you are feeling.
- *Your children.* Your children will notice that you are not yourself at some times of the month. Let them know that it is not their fault and explain what you *are* able to do for them. Children may not ask *why* things happen and presume that it is their fault. This is a burden they should not have to bear. There may be good things to come out of your illness. A mother who rests more and limits her social obligations is more available to cuddle or have quiet times with her children.
- *Your friends.* Over time, your friendships with some people may change. It is hard to maintain every friendship when your pain makes you cancel activities at the last moment, or cut down on

some social activities. Your friends may tire of asking how you are feeling. You can surround yourself with a few good friends who will support you no matter what. Be aware that your friends have troubles of their own. They may not have endometriosis, but we all have problems and there may be times when you can help them in some way. Even if this is difficult physically, you can still be a good listener. Friendships work best when there is listening and support on both sides. Your friends may be embarrassed to bring up their own troubles when your problems seem so much more important than theirs.

- *Your workmates.* All workplaces (and bosses) are different, but it may be sensible to tell them what is happening. You may prefer that your employer does not know about your condition, especially if you can cope with all your duties easily. However, if your pain is severe, they will notice your time off work, lack of concentration and inability to meet deadlines. If you have a reasonable boss, he or she will appreciate the effort you are making to get better and manage your pain. Without an explanation they might feel that you are not interested in your work. If you have an unreasonable boss, then you may be better to keep this information to yourself unless it becomes necessary to explain. If you feel that you are being mistreated because of your illness, your workplace representative or the Equal Opportunities Commission may be able to help you.

Feeling feminine and attractive

Pain, bleeding, bloating and the side effects of some medications can make you feel unattractive. Some women describe this feeling as 'living in an alien body'. Not surprisingly, your morale and self-worth may suffer. It is time to look after yourself, both physically and emotionally.

- *Talk to your partner if you can.* The longer you feel these things without explaining how you feel the harder they may be to discuss. If you feel uncomfortable doing this, you may prefer to talk to a good female friend.

- *Do activities you enjoy* that allow you to relax and feel good about yourself. A long hot bath with your favourite bath salts and music, a facial or body massage. A do-it-yourself facial, or manicure can be just as good if your budget is limited.
- *Wear something comfortable* that is not tight around your abdomen and makes you feel attractive.

Involving your family in your care

It is a good idea to take someone you feel comfortable with to your appointments with the gynaecologist. This special person could be your parent, husband, boyfriend, girlfriend, sister, or anyone you choose. Having them there will give you more confidence and will help them to understand what is happening to you. If you need surgery, this special person may be able to come with you when you are admitted to hospital and support you while you are waiting for your surgery.

Involving your family with your care helps in practical ways too. An involved family will be more likely to help rearrange your sport, dance or other commitments according to your menstrual cycle.

Feeling scared of surgery

It's normal to be anxious about an operation, but a pity if that anxiety stops you making good decisions about your health. Finding out as much as you can about what your operation involves may help you feel better. A visit to the hospital before your admission is a good idea. There will be less that is unknown and therefore less to worry about on the day.

Although it is impossible to know *exactly* what your doctor will find at the operation, or *exactly* what treatment you will need, you can find out what the possibilities are. There are many websites on endometriosis and a list of those we find most useful are on page 277. Ask your doctor any questions that are on your mind. You should never feel that your questions are silly. They are about what matters to you. Your doctor may have written information for you to take home and read. When you go into hospital, tell the nursing staff if you are nervous, and don't be embarrassed to ask questions. The nurses are there to help you too.

Finally, while it *is* true that the only reliable way of diagnosing endometriosis is with surgery, *you never have to have surgery.* As explained in Chapter 5 on page 46 endometriosis is not a life-threatening condition. Surgery should be a choice you make after considering the options you have. It may be a good choice in many cases, but it is never your only choice. Some of the choices available to you are explained in Chapter 7.

J am anxious and scared all the time

If you are very anxious or miserable, there may be something more going on. As a woman with pelvic pain, you have probably been through a lot over the last few years. None of this is good for your morale or self-esteem, and all of this can easily add up to feelings of isolation or depression.

If your worries are not being taken seriously and you know something is not right with your body or your emotions, ask for help from the doctor you feel most comfortable with. If you have prolonged feelings of sadness or you cry a lot, you may be depressed. There is no shame in seeking help and you can do so without your friends knowing.

Psychologists are professionals who help you by working out strategies for coping with your own feelings and life stresses. A psychiatrist is a doctor who specialises in the treatment of mental illness including depression. Your general practitioner may be able to help you themselves, but if not, he or she can advise you which type of professional might suit you best. You may also find the book *Coping with Endometriosis* by Robert Phillips and Glenda Motta useful (Avery, USA, 2000).

When sex is painful

If period pain was not enough, many women with endometriosis have painful intercourse. This is especially common in women whose endometriosis is near the pouch of Douglas or in the uterosacral ligaments that lie behind the uterus. Although painful sex is a problem for women of any age, it is particularly distressing for young women just starting their sexual life. Intercourse with their partner is an important part of their relationship. To find it painful is a great disappointment. With every attempt at intercourse there may be two or three days of pain, and yet the desire to bond emotionally with their partner remains. Ultimately, it is no wonder that many women avoid intercourse altogether, leaving their partner feeling rejected and unloved.

Removing endometriosis at an operation may cure your pain with intercourse completely, but sometimes the pain remains. If so, it may be due to:

* Anxiety about intercourse itself
* Painful nerve receptors in the pelvis that continue to cause pain even when the original problem has been treated (see Chapter 9, page 178)
* Pelvic muscles that have become painful and tight after years of pain
* Sexual abuse or other traumatic events in your life
* Negative attitudes to sex you may have learned as you grew up
* Seeing scary movies or images relating to sex
* Uncertainty about your sexuality
* Other physical reasons for pain.

A counsellor, especially a sex counsellor, can help with some of these problems, but you should also explain your symptoms to your doctor. Your general practitioner can check for physical reasons for the pain that may be nothing to do with your endometriosis (see Chapter 2, page 19). A sex counsellor can help bring up some of the topics you find most difficult to discuss with your partner, even if you choose to see the sex counsellor alone at first. They can help with:

- Exercises to improve your self-confidence and increase the trust between you and your partner
- Relaxation techniques
- Forms of sexual pleasure that are not painful
- Improving your communication skills as a couple
- Pain management
- Working out what works best for you.

But J just find it SO hard to talk to my partner about sex

Even close couples have some things they find hard to discuss, but it is important that you and your partner can communicate well. Men do not have pain that stops their sex drive, so without an explanation he will not understand. He may feel that you are avoiding sex because you no longer love him, rather than because sex is painful.

Misunderstandings that can damage your relationship happen easily. You may find it easier if your partner comes to your doctor's appointment with you. As your partner learns more about endometriosis and the effects it can have, your discussions about sex may become easier.

- Tell your partner what they do that does satisfy you, rather than presume they know already.

- Tell your partner that you still desire him (or her).
- Discuss your pain and tell him (or her) where it hurts.

  A healthy sexual relationship is important for both of you, so it is worth getting it right.

Avoiding pain during sex

Ideas for maintaining your sexual relationship despite pain include:

- *Working out which time of the day or month is least painful for you,* and arranging some special time together then. This often means having intercourse early in the month, just after your period, or early in the day when you are not tired.
- *Slow, shallow and gentle penetration until you say it is OK* allows you to stay in control. You will have more control of the depth of penetration if you are on top of your partner. Knowing that intercourse will not proceed further than you wish, allows you to feel more confident. Your partner will be fearful of hurting you so will appreciate a lead from you. A shorter time of penetration may avoid prolonged pain afterwards.
- *A water-based lubricant* such as KY Jelly, or Astroglide may make penetration easier. Natural lubrication only occurs if you are relaxed and pain free. This is a big ask of women with endometriosis, so it is not surprising that many use a lubricant. Many women without endometriosis use lubricants too, so there is no need to be embarrassed.
- *Relaxation techniques before sex.* Gentle and prolonged fore-play helps relax your pelvic muscles as well as giving you time to relax your whole body. Most women appreciate longer foreplay before penetrative sex. A pelvic physiotherapist can teach you how to strengthen your pelvic muscles, relax over-tight muscles or dilate an overly tight vagina.

- *New sexual positions.* The pain of endometriosis is usually worse in some positions than others.
- *Consider a medication* for neuropathic pain, such as amitriptyline (see Chapter 6, page 72). This is particularly useful in women with pain on most days of the month, or a 'burning' pain during intercourse.
- *Hypnotherapy* may be useful.

If penetration becomes impossible, you and your partner may be able to find other ways to pleasure each other. The book *Good Loving, Great Sex* by Rosie King (see Reference 27) has good suggestions for 'outercourse' rather than 'intercourse', as well as good ideas for mismatched sex drives.

Worries that you won't have children

Most women with endometriosis fear infertility. As explained in Chapter 8 on page 119, endometriosis is only one of several factors that can affect a couple's fertility. Endometriosis by itself does not mean you cannot become pregnant. A lot depends on how severe it is, where it is, how old you are, and whether there are other fertility issues present affecting either you or your partner. Almost all women with endometriosis are able to have children, even if some require medical assistance to do so.

If you do have difficulty becoming pregnant and are referred to a fertility specialist, there is usually a counsellor at the clinic with whom you can discuss your particular issues. Remember that your partner may have concerns of their own that they may find difficult to discuss with you. Now, more than ever, is the time when communication between you as a couple is so important. Yes, you are trying for a baby, but your relationship is important too. It is the two of you who matter most and a healthy relationship between you is important when caring for a child.

Not ready for a hysterectomy

Mandy is a woman in her late thirties who, although single, would love to have a child. Mandy has adenomyosis, a condition with pain similar to endometriosis due to changes in the wall of the uterus. Her doctor had offered her a hysterectomy and she was very distressed. Mandy knew that a hysterectomy would cure both her pain and the heavy bleeding she suffered, but she did not want to lose the chance of a pregnancy. We talked about her feelings and her yearnings to have a child one day. To avoid a hysterectomy, she needed strategies to help her cope with the pain.

Mandy decided to take one of the specialist's options and go on the contraceptive pill continuously to stop her periods and hopefully avoid her severe period pain. She would see a complementary therapist to help boost her immune system, and help with her general health and wellbeing. She would improve her diet and start some regular exercise. Just deciding on a plan made Mandy feel better. She felt back in control of her health. She hoped to manage her pain this way until either she met a partner with whom she could form a relationship and try to start a family, or she felt psychologically ready to have a hysterectomy.

Don't let premenstrual syndrome (PMS) make everything worse

Premenstrual syndrome is a collection of symptoms that some women notice in the days before a period. These symptoms may be emotional or physical and include:

- Greasy skin
- Fluid retention
- Decreased libido
- Irritability

- Sore breasts
- Backache
- Fatigue
- Depression.

Severe PMS seems very common in women with endometriosis. This makes the time before a period particularly difficult. Not only is there the pain of endometriosis, but the symptoms of PMS as well. The closer a period comes, the more anxiety a woman may feel. She knows the pain will come soon. Any PMS symptoms are the last straw.

Some women notice PMS symptoms for just one or two days before a period, while others suffer for up to two weeks. Women with mild symptoms may be able to carry on with their day-to-day life well despite their PMS, but for women with severe symptoms it can be debilitating. Severe PMS can contribute to accidents, antisocial behaviour, emotional crisis, and time off work or school. Stress does not cause PMS, but like most things, it makes it worse. In extreme cases, some women may feel suicidal.

While feeling forgetful or reclusive is common, aggression is the symptom that most women, their families and friends relate to most. There is also the guilt that women feel when they think about how their behaviour impacts on those closest to them.

If your symptoms are due to PMS, they will become worse the closer you are to a period. If they come at any time of the month, regardless of when your next period is due, then PMS is less likely, and you should talk to your general practitioner about it.

PMS just part of the problem

Mary and Rod have two small children. Rod worked long hours, with Mary as the main caregiver to their children, 24 hours a day, 7 days a week. Mary battled with her mood swings and her endometriosis pain. Rod suffered the mood swings too. Mary had no outlet and no close supportive family, so she rang Rod at work when she couldn't cope with the pain or the children. Rod's work suffered, as did their marriage. Their problems at times seemed monumental.

Mary and Rod felt better after we discussed what PMS and endometriosis involve, as well as Mary's feelings of loss of self, lack of support and entrapment with the children. Some strategies were put in place. Mary decided to have surgery to remove her endometriosis and lessen her pain. Once fully recovered she would look for a job outside the family. Rod would attempt to get home at a more reasonable hour to help with the children and support her plans to re-enter the workforce.

When I saw Mary again, she had started a part-time job that she enjoyed. She enjoyed her time with the children more now, and so did they. Working in the evening fitted in with both Rod and the children's needs. Her surgery had improved her pain and she felt much more positive about her life. So did Rod.

Ways that you can manage your PMS

- *Explain to your partner and family how your PMS affects you.* If you feel unable to do this, your counsellor or general practitioner may be able to help. An explanation that you have limited control over your emotions at that time, particularly if stressed, will ease family tension. They need to know that you need extra understanding at this time and are not 'putting it on'.

- *Manage your pain.* Your pain has not caused your PMS, but with less pain, you will have more energy to cope with your PMS. You will no longer dread the start of a period.

- *Improve your diet.* A diet that is low in salt (to reduce fluid retention), high in fibre and low in fat (to avoid bowel symptoms), high in fruits and vegetables (to supply the vitamins and minerals you need) and low in caffeine (to avoid over-stimulation) should suit you best.

- *Practice relaxation techniques* such as yoga, or meditation. Relaxation improves your ability to cope with PMS as well as allowing you 'time out' from the stress of family and work commitments. Time for relaxation allows you to regain control of your emotions.

- *Herbal therapies* (see Chapter 12). Natural therapists believe that PMS is due to an excess of oestrogen effect in the body. They use a combination of herbal therapies and diet to decrease the effect of oestrogen.

- *Exercise*. Exercise improves mental as well as physical well-being.

- *Consider trying the contraceptive pill.* The Pill improves many of the symptoms of PMS. It doesn't suit everyone, but can certainly help. Your doctor can help you decide if the Pill might suit you.

- *Consider an SSRI medication* (see Chapter 6, page 67). These medications stabilise a substance called serotonin in the brain. They can be useful for mood changes before your period. If your life is severely affected by your mood at this time, you may wish to discuss this medication with your general practitioner.

Remember, if your family is at breaking point because of your PMS, don't feel guilty: see your doctor or a family therapist. Help *is* available.

Coping once your treatment is finished

After you have spent a good deal of time seeing your GP, finding an endometriosis surgeon, having your surgery and working through other treatments, there comes a time when you come out of the treatment arena and return to your normal life. Until now you have been active in your treatment choices, but secure in the knowledge that others were there to care for you and help with decision making when needed. Some women find 'going it alone' a nervous and challenging time. *However, it is also an opportunity to be positive, grab hold of your life and move forward.*

Remember that if you need help your general practitioner is still there. He or she knows you well and is the best person to coordinate your long-term care. The relaxation techniques, dietary changes, exercise program, and whatever else has helped you become well should continue. If your symptoms return, your general practitioner can discuss your options with you and arrange an appointment with your specialist if necessary.

How your partner can support you and themselves

This book has concentrated on *her* needs, but *your* needs are important too. A healthy relationship values and provides support to both partners. At times one partner may need more care than the other, but if possible there should be mutual support. You may feel frustrated and resentful that her illness has impacted so much on your life. Even though your partner is in pain, your feelings are still there and still valid. You could talk to a friend about how you feel, take some time out that is just for you, see a counsellor yourself or plan things together that you *both* enjoy.

Telling other people about endometriosis

Endometriosis can be an embarrassing illness for a woman to have. It is much easier to explain an illness which is visible to the outside world (like a broken leg), an illness that will reliably get better over time (like pneumonia), or an illness that affects men too (like asthma or diabetes). It may be difficult or embarrassing for her to explain what her problem is to some friends, family or workmates. There may be some people she does not want to explain her endometriosis to at all.

Making her feel good about herself

When she feels unattractive, try to make her feel loved and desirable. Remember that she is often as confused about her feelings and the disease she is trying to cope with as you are. Flowers are good, but something practical to make her life easier, like a dinner cooked when she comes home, or an offer to get the kids off to school yourself may be even better. Often just an extra 'I love you' is all that is needed. Men rarely understand why women need repeated reassurance that they are loved and desirable. It is the way we women are. Be free with your kind comments. It is unlikely you will overdo it.

Deciding on a treatment option

It is difficult to be a partner of a woman with endometriosis. Men traditionally want to fix any problems their partners have. They want to save their partner from worry. You may feel powerless to help her when she has pain, and at a loss what to do. This is where the difference between men and women is an advantage. Most women neither expect nor want their man to come up with an answer to their problems. What they want is the opportunity to talk about and talk around their problems, sometimes at some length. This talking may seem unhelpful to a man, but it allows her to consider all aspects of the choices she has and come up with a considered and thoughtful plan that she is happy with. Listening to what she is thinking and how she feels is something very worthwhile that you *can* do. She will also want to know your views and ideas.

Helping her through her PMS

The lack of emotional control at this time distresses women and their families a lot. Women often say that 'they know they are being awful but just can't help it'. Then again, if you disregard what a woman says because 'it's that time of the month again' she may feel slighted and become even angrier. There is no need to tell her she is being unreasonable. She will feel bad enough later, when she recalls what she has said to those who love her most. Some ways in which you can support but not aggravate her include:

- *Giving her some time to herself*, to allow her to relax and get the things done which are on her mind.
- *Listening* if she wants to talk to you, but don't take insults to heart. During this time unexpected outbursts of anger or tears are common.
- *Encouraging her* to seek help for her symptoms, on a day when she feels well. Offer to go with her when she sees her doctor, counsellor or natural therapist, but allow her to go alone if she would prefer.
- *Helping her* work through any issues that trouble her, to relieve stress.
- *Recognising* that the time before a period is not a good time for her to make important decisions.
- *Avoiding* overloading her daily commitments at this time.

Coping with fertility treatment

For couples who *do* have difficulty becoming pregnant, there are new issues to consider. Certainly there is the grief that goes with not becoming pregnant easily, but there may also be concerns about:

- The lack of privacy over something that is usually so intimate
- The side effects of any medications used
- The expense of fertility treatments
- The increased chance of twins or triplets with some fertility treatments
- The rollercoaster of emotions associated with each pregnancy attempt

- The need to keep working for financial reasons (this may be true for both you and your partner)
- Coping with family, friends or workmates who constantly ask how things are going
- The loneliness of going through treatment that has been kept secret from family and friends
- The jealousy you feel when your partner's desire to have a child overtakes all other interests, including your relationship. You may feel guilty that you feel this way.

If you can, try to find a balance between the demands of your treatment and time for each other. It helps to make special time for each other that is not about baby making. If you have a very hectic working life, this is a good time to reduce your working hours and avoid over-committing yourself. You or your partner may not have the time or energy available to devote to a busy working life, your relationship *and* the demands of fertility treatment.

The desire to have children can be very strong, and even those who don't want to have children may feel distressed if the option to do so is lost. Choosing not to have a child feels very different from knowing that you no longer have the choice.

Some women who had never wanted children before change their mind as they get older. We are all entitled to change our mind over time, but this may be a problem for a couple whose relationship is based on a mutual desire to remain childless. The whole topic of fertility may become so emotional that it is impossible to discuss reasonably. This is where time with a counsellor or your general practitioner can help.

The men's website/newsletter at:

http://www.geocities.com/HotSprings/Spa/8449/eccpartners.html or, www.endometriosis.org.uk/partners

has useful information and support for you.

Not ready for a baby

Zena is a married woman in her mid-thirties. Zena had had painful periods for many years, and was considering a laparoscopy to look for endometriosis. The pain was severe, but Zena's biggest problem was her desire to have children. Up until now she and her husband had chosen not to have children. They had boats, motorbikes, a huge mortgage and two full-time jobs to give them the lifestyle they enjoyed. Their friends were childless by choice. We all change our mind sometimes and now Zena wanted a baby before it was too late.

Hugo had worries of his own. He had taken many years to decide to marry Zena. His previous marriage had failed and he was fearful of his marriage to Zena failing too. He was now fearful of pregnancy, and losing the lifestyle he loved.

Zena decided to have a laparoscopy to find out how severe her endometriosis was, and have it removed. This would help her pain, but also give her a better idea of how easily she might fall pregnant. Zena and Hugo needed help. Trying to discuss their differing needs themselves had only resulted in emotion, and conflict without resolution. Consulting a marriage counsellor could help. Involving a third person, acceptable to both people, might help them come to an arrangement that met both their needs.

Lesbian couples with fertility concerns

Lesbian couples may have similar problems to heterosexual couples, when it comes to fertility treatment. However, they may have other problems too:

- The legal availability of fertility services for same sex couples varies from country to country and state to state. You may need to travel away from home to access the services you need.

- To become pregnant, you will require semen from either a friend or an anonymous donor. You may be uncertain about the history of your donor, their personality, appearance, risk of genetic disease, or desire to contact your child later.
- Other people may not understand your desire for children and distress at infertility when you are in a same-sex relationship.
- There may be a lack of understanding if one of you has chosen to be the biological mother when the other partner is more fertile.
- Finding a support group suitable for your needs may be more difficult.

Then again, it will be easier for you to keep your sexual relationship separate to your quest for a baby.

Therapists and support groups

How to choose a good counsellor or complementary therapist

There is a wide range of therapists available, so this can be a bewildering decision.

The first thing to decide on is the type of practitioner you are looking for. You may be comfortable with some types of therapy but not others. Your general practitioner or specialist may recommend a therapist with whom they work regularly, but not all therapists suit all women so you may need to find a therapist yourself.

The next thing to decide is what you are looking for from this therapist.

- What symptoms do I wish them to treat?
- Does this therapist have recognised qualifications in their special area? Most qualified practitioners will belong to a professional organisation.

- Are they happy to work together with your doctor? If not, you may find yourself with two conflicting sets of advice.
- Will it be a long wait for an appointment? In some cases it will be worth the wait. In others there may be another person you could see instead.
- What are the costs involved, and are these costs covered by the NHS or private insurance? Do they charge for missed appointments?
- What time of the day or day of the week are appointments available?
- Will the possibility of treatment by a person of a different ethnic origin or gender be a problem for you?
- What sort of techniques do they use?
- Will there be a set time for treatment and the opportunity to discuss progress and change track if necessary?

Once you have met with your therapist, ask yourself whether you felt comfortable with that person and the treatment he or she recommended. Did you feel confident that that person had *your* best interests at heart? Did you feel able to communicate with them, and was your point of view listened to and acknowledged? Did the treatment recommended make sense and are you happy to go ahead with it? If not, it is not too late to go elsewhere. Most treatment programs require dedication and commitment, so if you are not comfortable with the treatment offered, it is less likely to be successful.

There are no easy fixes for pelvic pain so it is important that you and your therapist are able to build a good honest working relationship. Whatever treatment path you decide on, ask your practitioner how long it will be before you should see improvement. Some treatments do not work instantly, and may need time, but you don't want to waste time on something that just isn't working for you.

> ## Feel optimistic!
>
> There are many reasons why you can feel optimistic despite the problems that you have. Endometriosis is now recognised as a significant problem for many women. You are certainly not alone. The ways to diagnose endometriosis are improving and treatment options are now more effective. Research into even better ways to manage endometriosis continues. If you have older relatives with severe endometriosis, it is unlikely that you will suffer as they have. A lot has improved. Things are better now.

Finding an endometriosis support group

Most endometriosis support groups are made up of women who have had endometriosis themselves. It is very comforting to be among other women with similar experiences. However, support is a very individual thing and different women look for different things in a support group. You should consider:

- What sort of support do I need?
- Can the support group support me in this way, or should I see a psychologist or psychiatrist?
- Does attending my support group give me a positive experience?
- Is the support group well run?
- Where are meetings held? Is this a convenient place for me and do I feel comfortable with the surroundings?
- Would I prefer anonymous support, possibly by phone or email?

Support groups around the world

Britain

Contact either The National Endometriosis Society:

Address: 50 Westminster Palace Gdns, Artillery Row, London
             SW1P 1RR
Phone: 020 7222 2781
Email: nes@endo.org.uk
Website: www.endo.org.uk

or The Endometriosis SHE Trust (UK):

Address: 14 Moorland Way, Lincoln LN6 7JW
Phone: 08707 743665
Email: shetrust@shetrust.org.uk
Website: www.shetrust.org.uk

Australia
Contact the Endometriosis Association of Victoria:

Phone: (03) 9870 0536, (03) 9827 2199 or (03) 9457 2933
Website: www.endometriosis.org.au
Email: info@endometriosis.org.au
Support Line: 1800 069 697 (toll free in Victoria)

New Zealand
Contact the New Zealand Endometriosis Foundation:

Address: PO Box 1673, Mail Centre, Christchurch
Phone: 03 379 7959
Website: www.nzendo.co.nz
Email: nzendo@xtra.co.nz

United States of America
Contact the Endometriosis Research Center:

Address: 630 Ibis Drive Delray Beach, FL 33444 USA
Phone: 800/239 - 7280 (Toll Free) or 561/274-0931
Fax: 561/274-0931
Website: www.endocenter.org

Chapter 12

. . . .

Complementary medicine for endometriosis

Dr Margaret Taylor

NATURAL OR 'COMPLEMENTARY' MEDICINE offers some fascinating ideas for the treatment of endometriosis and these ideas work well in conjunction with conventional medicine and surgery. If the body is well nourished by a healthy and appropriate diet and supplemented with vitamins, minerals and herbs, it will be much better equipped to deal with surgery and medical drugs. It is also better able to deal with side effects from such treatments. That is why natural medicine is now often called complementary medicine, because it complements conventional medicine.

The body always tries to heal itself, and sometimes all it needs to recover from a problem is the correct food and environment. Many people have heard of someone who has unexpectedly recovered from a serious illness, such as cancer for example, and surprised everyone. There is no one reason for such a recovery. It usually means that many elements of the treatment contributed to such a healing. Often the first thing to consider is improving lifestyle and diet, both of which today are a long way from being 'natural'.

The body is an intricate system that relies on all parts for it to work effectively, just as a team does. Relieving a symptom is often not possible unless you fix the underlying problem. This is why complementary medicine takes a holistic approach to illness, looking at the whole system because there is rarely one pill or treatment that will work without the patient changing to a healthier way of life that benefits the whole body.

The complementary approach to endometriosis

There seem to be three important differences between the endometriosis lesions in the abdomen and the normal endometrial lining in the uterus:

- Women with endometriosis have relatively too much oestrogen
- Endometriosis lesions contain aromatase, the enzyme that makes oestrogen
- There is inflammation around the lesions, which usually means a sufferer will feel pain.

These factors come together in a damaging self-perpetuating cycle where inflammation stimulates aromatase, which produces oestrogen, which in turn increases inflammation. Sounds hard? Just look at the diagram (Figure 12.1).

Fortunately there are a lot of natural treatments that slow the cycle down, and most of them you can manage yourself, although some medications need a prescription. In this chapter we will look at the natural controls of this cycle and consider how it can be influenced by foods and natural supplements. There are many

Figure 12.1 The endometriosis cycle

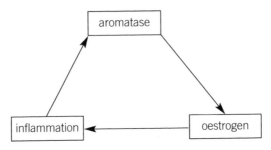

factors involved and it may seem complicated, but taken one at a time they are all quite simple. I find that people like to know why they have to take a particular supplement or food. You generally feel more powerful and in control if you understand why something happens. If it seems too complicated, there is a summary and an eating plan at the end of the chapter.

Oestrogen and endometriosis

In complementary medicine it is considered that the main problem in endometriosis is *oestrogen dominance.*

Oestrogen dominance is a common condition these days, where there is relatively too much oestrogen, especially compared to its partner hormone — progesterone. It can result in sore lumpy breasts (fibrocystic breast disease), painful periods (dysmenorrhoea), premenstrual syndrome (PMS) and endometriosis.

The causes of oestrogen dominance
- Slow breakdown of oestrogen by the liver
- Increased conversion of testosterone to oestrogen by the enzyme aromatase
- Decreased plant oestrogens (phyto-oestrogens) in your diet
- Xeno-oestrogens (toxic chemicals that behave like oestrogen) in food, air and water.

To reduce oestrogen dominance

- Reduce the fat in your diet
- Lose weight
- Introduce friendly (probiotic) bacteria to your gut
- Increase phyto-oestrogens in your diet
- Undergo liver detoxification
- Reduce caffeine
- Exercise
- Increase natural progesterone
- Try a herb, vitex agnus castus (also called 'chaste tree')
- Avoid xeno-oestrogens
- Block aromatase with zinc, herbs or chrysin.

How can J know if J have too much oestrogen?

You might have painful, swollen or even lumpy breasts, nausea, fluid retention and abdominal bloating, heavy periods, fatigue, weight gain, craving for sweets and/or premenstrual irritability and depression.

Reducing the fat in your diet

Oestrogen is normally broken down in the liver and then excreted into the bowel. However, eating saturated animal fats encourages the growth of intestinal bacteria, which produce an enzyme called beta-glucuronidase. This enzyme converts it back into a form that can be reabsorbed. So oestrogen can cycle round and round between the gut, the bloodstream and the liver many times before it is finally excreted!

This means that women (and men) who eat more animal fat have significantly higher levels of oestrogen than those on low fat diets. A high animal fat intake has been linked with benign breast cysts, breast cancer, heavy menstruation, endometriosis, fibroids and prostate enlargement in men. All these conditions are thought to relate to high oestrogen. Other research has actually shown that reducing your fat intake leads to lower oestrogen in the body.

How do I reduce the fat in my diet?

A low fat diet means reducing foods such as butter, margarine, ice cream and cheese as well as the visible fat on meat. Fried foods are particularly high in fat. Don't reduce the good fats, which are found in foods such as avocado, olive oil, nuts and seeds.

What is Calcium D-glucarate?

Calcium D-glucarate is a special supplement that stops the beta-glucuronidase in the bowel from remaking oestrogen after it has been broken down in the liver and, in my clinical experience, it can be effective in lowering oestrogen. It is available in the USA (500 mg capsules) and can usually be imported into other countries for personal use. It is also found in small amounts in spinach, carrots and apples.

Lose weight

Fat cells contain the enzyme aromatase, so people who are obese make more oestrogen. The type of obesity may be important. Apple shaped women with a high waist measurement, tend to have high *insulin* levels. Insulin regulates the amount of sugar in the blood and is discussed on page 261. They have more free oestrogen than pear shaped women with the weight in the thighs. Apple shaped women (with most of the weight around the middle) probably won't be able to lose weight on a low fat diet. A low carbohydrate diet which reduces insulin would be much more effective. (This is discussed in insulin reduction on page 261.) Regardless of the diet you follow, it is essential to eat lots of vegetables, which are mostly low in carbohydrates and high in fibre and antioxidants. (See the Eating Plan on page 269.)

Why should J eat more vegetables?

High fibre, low fat diets can reduce the activity of the enzyme beta-glucuronidase so less oestrogen is able to re-enter the bloodstream. Vegetables, fruit, legumes (beans and lentils), muesli, wholemeal bread and wholemeal pasta are high in fibre and low in fat. They are high in antoxidants and other food chemicals that prevent various cancers, by reducing damage to DNA.

Introducing friendly (probiotic) bacteria to your gut

Yoghurt has bacteria like lactobacillus acidophilus, which reduce the production of beta-glucuronidase, that enzyme that remakes oestrogen. Eating yoghurt is associated with a lower incidence of breast cancer (see Reference 28) possibly by reducing the re-absorption of oestrogen or by enhancing the immune system. It should also be good for endometriosis. It must be yoghurt with a live culture, rather than just any yoghurt. If you are allergic to milk (see allergies page 260), use soy milk or take capsules of acidophilus.

Eating more phyto-oestrogens

Phyto-oestrogens are plant hormones that behave just like weak oestrogens. All cells have oestrogen receptors — brain, skin, uterus, and even endometriosis cells. A receptor is like a lock and oestrogen is the key that fits in the lock and turns on certain processes in the cell. Phyto-oestrogens are amazing substances –

they act like oestrogen but are hundreds of times less active than oestrogen. When they occupy the oestrogen receptor they prevent some of the normal oestrogen from affecting the cell. This means that where there is too much oestrogen, such as in endometriosis, phyto-oestrogens can reduce the effectiveness of normal oestrogen; but where there is not enough oestrogen, after menopause for example, they can behave like weak oestrogen and help prevent hot flushes and loss of bone density.

Most traditional diets, for example Mediterranean, African and Asian diets, contain many more phyto-oestrogens than the Western diet and it is thought that this is why those people have less oestrogen-related cancer. Phyto-oestrogens are found mainly in legumes, such as soy products (tofu, tempeh, soy milk), beans, lentils, peas, and chickpeas, that are commonly deficient in a Western diet. To increase phyto-oestrogens in your system, add foods such as baked beans, bean salads, lentil soups and patties, hummus, as well as soy linseed bread to your diet. Try adding tinned beans to all your curries and casseroles. If you are worried about wind, start slowly. Eat only small amounts at first and gradually build up, having a little each day. As the bacteria in the intestines get used to these foods, the problem should settle.

Linseed – another natural oestrogen blocker

Linseed contains high amounts of lignans, which block oestrogen receptors in the cell and reduce its effect. Three teaspoons a day of ground linseed, or a mix often referred to as LSA – ground linseed, sesame seeds and almonds – on your vegetables or cereal should be enough.

The cabbage family and oestrogen

The cabbage family vegetables should be consumed regularly by women who have oestrogen-related conditions. They include all cabbages, broccoli, kale, bok choy, cauliflower, brussels sprouts and radicchio. Substances called 'indoles' found in these vegetables seem to increase the breakdown of oestrogen in a way that reduces breast cancer cell growth. These indoles are available as supplements of di-indolyl methane or indole-3-carbinol from natural practitioners if there is a problem eating enough of these vegetables. The herb rosemary also helps in this way. You could make a weak tea and drink it three times a day.

Liver detoxification

Foods high in sulphur, like beans, legumes, onions and garlic help the liver break down oestrogen. The same processes that are used to excrete toxic chemicals also break down oestrogen, so there can be a bottleneck at times, and naturopaths describe this by saying the liver is 'stressed'. The diagnostic methods used by naturopaths can often pick this up before a blood test for liver function test (LFT) is abnormal, because the LFT picks up liver cell damage, not poor function. Some herbs are useful for improving liver function. These include St Mary's thistle, dandelion and globe artichoke. Many liver detox formulas combine the above herbs with some antioxidants to protect the liver cells. A good liver formula would also have some sulphur-containing amino acids such as methionine, choline, inositol, and taurine.

Additional vitamin C is also useful — 1000 mg per day or more and it can be continued long term.

Cutting down on caffeine

Drinking 4–5 cups of coffee a day increases oestrogen by nearly 70 per cent. Tea has about half as much caffeine. Decaffeinated tea or coffee or herbal tea would be a good alternative to help keep oestrogen as low as possible.

Exercise

Exercise helps with oestrogen clearance, and women who exercise tend to have lower oestrogen levels, lighter and less frequent periods. It also reduces insulin resistance, which makes it easier to lose weight (see page 262). The exercise doesn't have to be extreme — walking, cycling or swimming for 20–30 minutes, four or five times a week, is sufficient, and exercising in the morning is even better. If small children or other responsibilities prevent you getting out for a walk or to the gym, an exercise bike can be useful. Put it in front of the TV and pedal away, or turn on the early morning television aerobics program. For those suffering pelvic pain, the bike may be less painful than other exercises because the pelvis does not bounce when you use the bike.

Natural progesterone

This is an important natural treatment for endometriosis. Progesterone is produced by the ovary after ovulation and naturally balances the effects of oestrogens. Some women don't produce enough. This can happen because of stress, or peri-menopause, or from toxic chemicals called xeno-oestrogens (see page 257).

Progesterone has some pleasant effects. It is probably the reason that women look and feel so good in later pregnancy. It matures the endometrium each month to prevent heavy periods, and has many effects all over the body that include:

- Helping us use fat for energy
- Helping thyroid hormone
- Being a natural anti-depressant
- Being a natural diuretic
- Normalising blood sugar levels
- Restoring libido (sexual appetite)
- Protecting against breast fibrocysts and helping prevent breast cancer

- Helping prevent endometrial cancer
- Being necessary for the survival of an embryo
- Stimulating the cells that make bone.

Natural progesterone cream rubbed into thin skin is well absorbed. It can only be obtained with a prescription from a doctor. Look around for one who is familiar with its use. In the USA you can buy progesterone cream over the counter as it is very safe. Progesterone in the body can be monitored by measuring levels in saliva, as it is not detected on a blood test when administered in a skin cream.

The normal progesterone script is either a 1.5 or 3 per cent cream. Higher doses may be required for pain management in endometriosis. In fact, levels around about 54–60 mg (5–6 per cent progesterone cream) may be necessary and appear to be well tolerated. Symptoms of excess progesterone are sleepiness and sluggishness and most women will find that they can or should reduce their dosage of progesterone after a few months. However, attempts to go below, say, 4 per cent progesterone (40 mg/gm cream) may allow symptoms to recur. You may get *oestrogenic* symptoms at first, so it helps to have a doctor who can guide you, so you don't give up too soon. It can be used in conjunction with the Pill as it does not interfere with the contraceptive effect, and it should help with some of the side effects as well as possibly reducing the endometriosis.

I have been unable to find any reliable research on the results of using natural progesterone in endometriosis, but one doctor who is using it has said that 75 per cent of his endometriosis patients get some relief (Reference 29). Dr John Lee, who popularised natural progesterone cream, stated that it is very effective for mild to moderate endometriosis, but further solid research is needed to prove it one way or the other.

What is the difference between natural progesterone, wild yam extract and progestins?

Natural progesterone is made in the corpus luteum of the ovary after ovulation (20–25 mg per day) and by the placenta during pregnancy (up to 300–400 mg/day — an astonishing increase). Wild yam extract is not a progesterone. It actually has an oestrogenic effect! Progestins are sometimes referred to as progesterone, but they are only synthetic versions of it. Although, like progesterone, they are useful for preventing heavy bleeding in the uterus, in other areas of the body (such as the brain) they can interfere with natural progesterone and can cause PMS or depression.

Vitex agnus castus (chaste tree)

Vitex is a useful herb for many women as it encourages the ovary to ovulate more effectively and produce more of its own natural progesterone from the corpus luteum after ovulation. Many research studies in Europe have shown its effectiveness for simple period pain and premenstrual syndrome, and it's an important herb for endometriosis. Use 500–1000 mg in the morning. This won't work if you are on the contraceptive pill, because the Pill prevents ovulation.

Avoid xeno-oestrogens

Many modern chemicals are xeno-oestrogens. They include pesticides, plasticisers, alkylphenols, PCBs, dioxins, cadmium and lead. They are similar enough to oestrogen to mimic its action in the body. The difficult thing about these chemicals is that they seem to be everywhere. Reproductive disorders such as sterility are occurring in wildlife, and girls are maturing sexually much earlier than before. These may be effects due to xeno-oestrogens. We all have xeno-oestrogen in our bodies. For example, nine healthy volunteers in New York in 2003 had an average of 91 industrial chemicals in their body, some of which were xeno-oestrogens. These people do not live in a toxic area or work with chemicals. Xeno-oestrogens are very difficult for the body to eliminate, and are mainly found in the fatty tissues, and not much in the watery part of the blood, so blood tests don't give a true picture.

Dioxins are contaminants of weedicide 245T and by-products of industrial processes. They are the main toxic chemicals that have been researched for endometriosis. Monkeys who were given dioxin in their food (like us) for four years developed endometriosis spontaneously. Ten years later laparoscopy showed that the monkeys who received higher exposure to dioxins had developed more severe cases of the disease. By then their blood levels had come down to normal human levels (Reference 30). It seems that these chemicals can induce endometriosis and then it keeps going on its own, perhaps because of the self-perpetuating cycle described at the beginning of this chapter. In humans it is impossible to do this sort of research and the dioxins we are exposed to are so numerous that it is difficult to know which ones to measure in the blood. We do know that dioxins are more commonly found in the blood of women with endometriosis than women who don't have it. If you want to read more about xeno-oestrogens go to http://www.ewg.org/reports/bodyburden

How can I avoid xeno-oestrogens?

Pesticides can be minimised by eliminating them from your home and garden as far as possible, and by buying certified organic foods. If you're in areas commonly sprayed with pesticides (for example golf courses), take care to keep your hands away from your mouth and wash your hands thoroughly after exposure.

Pesticides are very easily absorbed through the skin.

Heavy metals such as cadmium and lead are also suspected xeno-oestrogens. Blood levels of lead are dropping in most people since the introduction of lead-free petrol, but some old houses have a huge lead burden in the dust and soil, mostly due to old lead paint. Cadmium can be found in superphosphate from Nauru and is now on lots of farmland, but it is also found in areas where industrial waste was dumped. There are apparently over 600 known toxic waste sites in Australia, many of them in areas that are now residential housing, so if you suspect that you have only been ill since moving to a certain house, you could find out the history of your land and/or get your soil analysed.

Plasticisers, for example phthalates, are used to help keep PVC plastic flexible in products such as toys, teething rings, shower curtains, floor coverings, car seats and some food wraps. Avoid them and reduce absorption by having plenty of fresh air in the house and car.

Other xeno-oestrogens include alkylphenols (in shampoo and cosmetics), bisphenol (a hardener in paints or lacquers such as the lining in tinned foods), or plastics (such as water pipes or bottle top linings). *Choice* magazine, October 1997, has further details.

Persistent organic pollutants. This group of chemicals has the most hormone-disrupting effects — it includes polychlorinated biphenols (PCBs), dioxins and some pesticides such as DDT. They have a long life, and they're widespread in the environment. Because they're fat-soluble, they're found especially in animal fat, so changing to organically grown meat and dairy foods will reduce exposure.

What if I can't reduce my exposure?

If you can't reduce exposure, the answer is to improve liver function to get rid of them more quickly. See the above section on liver clearance of oestrogen (page 253). We use the same processes to get rid of these chemicals. Onions, garlic and eggs have plenty of sulphur, which we need for excreting these toxic substances. (Sulphur is not the same as sulpha antibiotics.) Nature's phyto-oestrogens also help to reduce their effects — another reason to eat those beans! There is some research showing that excreting them through the skin by sweating is effective (Reference 31). So, showering after exercise or saunas and washing the skin with soap is worthwhile in conjunction with the liver formula and vitamin C.

Blocking aromatase

Aromatase is the enzyme that produces oestrogen from testosterone. As described on page 85 one of the most distinct things about endometriosis lesions is that the cells produce aromatase and normal endometrium doesn't.

Chrysin is a natural inhibitor of aromatase. It is a bioflavonoid from a plant. Chrysin was first used in the 1930s as part of breast cancer treatment and in 1993 (Reference 32) was shown to be similar in effectiveness to an aromatase-inhibiting drug (amino-glutethimide). It is now mainly used by men who want to stop all their testosterone being converted to oestrogen as they get older. It does the same in women — slows the conversion of androgens (testosterone) to oestrogen.

A great advantage of using plant extracts instead of pharma-ceuticals is that the plant extracts have other health benefits. Chrysin is also a potent antioxidant with vitamin-like effects in the body. It also has an anti-inflammatory effect, possibly by blocking the enzymes that make prostaglandins (see Chapter 6, page 64). These are both useful effects for women with endometriosis. As chrysin is poorly absorbed orally, it is not effective in tablet form. However, it can now be administered in a skin cream with excellent results. Chrysin is only available on prescription from a compounding pharmacy. 1 gm/day of 0.5 per cent cream is the correct dose for women.

Other natural inhibitors of aromatase include the herbs *epilobium*, *nettle* and *saw palmetto*, and the mineral *zinc*. They can all slow down the production of oestrogen by aromatase.

Inflammation and endometriosis

What is inflammation?

It's just the same as the hot red painful swelling that accompanies the healing of an injury or infection. The inflammation that occurs in the endometriosis lesions may be the cause of the pain of endometriosis. Unfortunately, high levels of oestrogen stimulate the COX enzyme to produce more prostaglandins (see Figure 6.1, page 65).

What increases inflammation (apart from oestrogen)?

Meat, fat and sugar are the simple answer. Meat and fat contain the arachidonic acid that prostaglandins are made from. Sugar is a problem because the excess amounts that are eaten these days stimulate *insulin resistance*, which is very inflammatory (see page 261). Blood in the peritoneal cavity can cause inflammation and may be why excess reflux of menstrual blood up the fallopian tubes may contribute to endometriosis.

Can food allergies affect inflammation?

Many people have undiagnosed food allergies that cause chronic problems such as sinusitis, tiredness, depression, an irritable bowel, eczema etc. If you have these symptoms as well as your endometriosis, it would help to find out and avoid the foods that are causing it, because they may be increasing inflammation. If your symptoms are mainly in the bowel, ask your doctor for a blood test for endomysial antibodies and gliadin antibodies because gluten in wheat and other grains are commonly the cause. If it's mainly sinus and mucus in the throat, try having *ABSOLUTELY* no milk or dairy products for a week and then have a glass of milk. This technique of eliminating something from the diet and then reintroducing it is the most accurate way of finding an answer, but eliminating the food properly can be difficult. Reading food labels is essential because, for example, bread can have milk in it. A nutritional doctor, naturopath or dietician would be able to guide you.

How can I reduce inflammation?

There are many ways to reduce inflammation:

- Reduce insulin resistance
- Eat more fish oil – more fish in your diet, or 1000 mg three times daily
- Anti-inflammatory herbs
- Other natural supplements such as Bromelain and Quercetin.

Insulin resistance

Eating foods with sugar causes the pancreas to produce insulin. When it happens excessively this condition is called *insulin resistance*. It increases the risk of heart disease and breast cancer. Insulin increases the amount of food going into the fat cells and makes it difficult to get it out again for energy. This is a major cause of putting on weight and leads to diabetes. Fat cells also produce oestrogen with the aromatase enzyme. Insulin also strongly increases inflammatory prostaglandins, so one of the most important ways to reduce pain would be to stop eating sugar and other carbohydrates such as pasta, rice, potato, many breakfast cereals, white bread, cake and biscuits with a high glycemic index (GI). High GI foods put the blood sugar up quickly which overstimulates insulin to reduce it again.

Insulin resistance can be reversed by exercising and eating like a modern hunter-gatherer. This means plenty of protein and vegetables and less starch and sugar. 10,000 years ago humans had no bread or pasta at all in their diet and were perfectly healthy, so don't worry that you'll miss out if you reduce them substantially. But you do need to eat lots of vegetables to ensure adequate fibre. The Atkins diet would be too inflammatory for women with endometriosis because there is too much red meat and fat and cream. There are other more healthy low carbohydrate diets with more vegetables and healthier fats and oils, for example the Zone diet or Protein Power. Exercise also reduces insulin resistance.

Fish and fish oils
Eat as much fish as possible — say 3–5 times a week. Increasing vegetables and fish increases the *Omega 3 fatty acids* that are nature's anti-inflammatories. The big fish such as shark/flake, ray, swordfish, barramundi, gemfish, orange roughy, ling and southern bluefin tuna accumulate lots of mercury because they are large, live longer, and are at the top of the food chain. You don't need to eliminate them altogether, but it's better to eat other smaller fish most of the time. Freshwater fish in geothermal lakes and rivers in New Zealand may also accumulate higher levels of mercury. Canned tuna has lower levels of mercury than fresh bluefin tuna because the tuna fish used for canning is a different, smaller species and is generally caught when less than 1 year old. Fish oils have Omega 3 fatty acids that inhibit endometriosis in laboratory research. One group of 50 women with endometriosis and gut pain, treated with a diet with less sugar, coffee and cheese and addition of olive oil and omega 3 fatty acids, improved significantly (Reference 34).

Herbs
There are some very effective herbs that inhibit inflammation. *Boswellia, devil's claw, turmeric* and *ginger* have all been shown to

possess similar anti-inflammatory activity to NSAIDs in arthritis (Reference 35). They reduce the production of prostaglandins, so there's no reason why they wouldn't work in endometriosis as well. The quality of herbal tablets and extracts can vary widely so it is better to get herbs from a herbalist, who can access top quality products from one of the herbal manufacturers who assay their products to make sure they are correct potency. These manufacturers often make a tablet combination of anti-inflammatory herbs that are much easier to take than herbal liquids. On the other hand, the advantage of using herbal liquids is that a good herbalist can combine herbs with different actions for your specific symptoms. The most common ones you might be given include:

- Cramp bark or dong quai for period pain
- Sedative or tonic herbs for stress
- St John's wort for depression
- Pulsatilla for ovarian pain
- Gotu kola or dan shen to reduce adhesions
- Vitex agnus castus to increase your progesterone
- Liver herbs (St Mary's thistle, globe artichoke, dandelion) to assist excretion of oestrogen and toxic chemicals
- Grapeseed extract or other powerful herbal antioxidants
- Nettle, epilobium or saw palmetto (pygeum) to inhibit aromatase.

Other natural supplements

Bromelain is an extract of pineapple, which has an anti-inflammatory effect similar to prednisone (a form of cortisone). Sports people use it to reduce bruising. The effective dose is 600–1200 mg per day.

Quercetin is a natural substance in foods especially tea, apples and onions. It is strongly anti-inflammatory and antioxidant. The effective dose would be 200–2000 mg/day. You can get 10–20 mg/day from foods.

Premenstrual syndrome

Will vitex help my PMS?

Probably/almost certainly. Some of my patients report the benefit within days! Almost always within the first month. Before I knew about vitex, I prescribed evening primrose oil and vitamin B6 and magnesium for PMS. They often helped a little, which is what the research says — some benefit, but not much.

- Vitex agnus castus — 1000 mg daily in the morning
- Vitamin B6 — 100 mg in the morning combined with a multivitamin and magnesium 400 mg daily
- Evening primrose oil — 1000 mg capsules 2 or 3 times daily. While vitex helps most women with PMS, evening primrose oil helps some but not others.

If vitex doesn't help you within the first month or two of treatment, your PMS may be related to too many sugar and milk products. Women with PMS eat more dairy products than other women — we don't know why. It would be worth a trial month off sugar and dairy foods to see if it helps you.

Vitamin B6 deficiency makes tissues in the uterus and breast more susceptible to the stimulating effects of oestrogen, and in my clinical experience, vitamin B6 deficiency is fairly common. Vitamin B6 should always be taken with other B vitamins and, as it gives some people vivid dreams, it should be taken in the morning. No more than 200 mg per day should be taken as it can cause nerve damage in high doses.

What if I feel as if I have PMS all month?

Tired, depressed, achy, irritable, bloated? If it happens in the first half of the month, it's not (just) PMS. It may be a food intolerance or allergy, especially if you have good and bad days. These foods are very addictive — 'milkaholics' may need milk many times a day, for example in coffee, and after a few days on a completely milk-free diet, they suddenly feel completely different — light, energetic, cheerful. They say, 'I never knew other people felt like this in the morning. It is so great to wake up with energy and enthusiasm for the day. And I'm not craving my coffee (with milk) all the time. I miss the milk in my coffee but it's worth it, to feel this good.' It could be any food you eat often, such as wheat, yeast, egg, tomato, sugar and so on. Find out by strictly eliminating the food you suspect from your diet for 10–14 days and then trying it. The result will be an obvious return of your symptoms if that particular food is causing the symptoms.

What about period pain?

As explained in Chapter 2, on page 13, not all period pain is endometriosis. Ordinary period pain will not respond as well as other symptoms to excisional surgery for endometriosis.

Here is where high tech medicine and natural remedies can work well together. Natural therapies for period pain include:

- Vitex agnus castus. This herb helps period pain because it increases the progesterone that matures the lining of the uterus, so it is released easily at period time
- Zinc 20–30 mg per day
- If these don't prevent it, try magnesium 200 mg every 2 hours while you have the cramps (Reference 36).

This is an email I got from a friend of mine who is a physiotherapist. 'Just a quick thank you for the vitex tip. Marked improvement this month in my period pain, so THANK YOU!!' She had only been on it 3 weeks!

Zinc

I learnt about zinc from one of my secretaries many years ago. She was typing a letter I'd written about zinc for another problem, which she also had, and decided to try it. She was amazed to find that her next period arrived with no pain. So was I, so I tried it on lots of other women and it often worked. Zinc deficiency is very common in women, and it is important for making hormones. In Australia a study has shown that 85 per cent of women do not get enough zinc in the food they eat (Reference 37) and most women with endometriosis would be in that 85 per cent. Zinc is in oysters, meat, fish, nuts, dried peas and beans. We need 11–15 mg/day when we are healthy, and probably twice that amount if we are not well. Supplements are safe to take even if you are not deficient, as long as you follow the directions. I suggest 30–50 mg/day, for example you might take zinc chelate 220 mg twice a day, because each tablet has about 20 mg of real zinc. In some brands this would be labelled 20 mg zinc (as chelate).

How can J know if J am deficient in zinc?

If you are deficient in zinc, you may have:
- White spots on your nails
- Poor wound healing and wound infection
- Slow growth and sexual maturation (late onset of periods)
- Poor appetite (anorexia) and taste disorder
- Poor resistance to infection.

Magnesium

Magnesium is nature's antispasmodic mineral. People who are low in magnesium can have restless legs, insomnia, anxiety, twitches in muscles, palpitations, leg cramps or period pain. If you are low in magnesium, then magnesium supplementation may help your period pain (Reference 37). But of course if your period pain has another cause, it won't help. Magnesium is in green vegetables, nuts and seeds. It is the middle of the chlorophyll molecule — the green pigment in plants that has the magical property of using sunlight, air and water to make the substance of plants. According to CSIRO research, 39 per cent of Australian women do not eat enough magnesium in their food (Reference 37).

How can J tell if J have magnesium deficiency?

Magnesium deficiency can cause:

- Restless legs
- Insomnia
- Anxiety
- Twitches in muscles
- Palpitations
- Leg cramps
- Period pain
- Heart attack.

Should I be on the Pill?

There is no simple answer to this question. The pain and disability of endometriosis can be significant and any relief possible is a great boon and should not be shunned for minor reasons. In natural medicine, barrier methods of contraception are preferred — diaphragms and condoms, but for some people the only practical contraception is the Pill. My opinion is that the research shows that it is a fairly benign medicine — even the long-term studies show little risk, especially when compared to other risks of modern life. So my suggestion is to use the Pill where necessary for symptomatic relief, and when symptoms improve you may be able to stop using it if you wish, or continue if you want to use it for contraception. The main question is whether you tolerate it well. There are many studies that show that nutrient needs are greater on the Pill, so it makes sense to take a multivitamin as well. The increased risk of breast cancer is *tiny* compared to the greatly increased risk due to smoking, alcohol or not exercising.

What about alcohol?

The effects of alcohol on oestrogen metabolism and oestrogen-related disorders are complex. Moderate alcohol consumption (one glass of beer, one glass of wine or one shot of spirits daily) has been associated with reduced levels of oestrogen (but an increased risk of breast cancer). Women who consume alcohol have a 50 per cent increase in risk of endometriosis. When the pain is bad, women with endometriosis tend to drink more alcohol. This is not the time to drink more alcohol as it increases inflammation and will only increase the pain. At other times a little (perhaps a glass or two a week) is probably OK.

Insomnia?

Do you have trouble sleeping or do you find that winter depresses you? You may be low in *melatonin*. This hormone helps us sleep and is important in preventing cancer. It also inhibits cyclo-oxygenase production of prostaglandins. Being exposed to bright light in the morning causes melatonin to be produced at bedtime. It decreases with ageing and is a popular anti-ageing supplement in the USA. Why not make sure your melatonin production is optimal by going for a walk in the morning? Homeopathic melatonin is available; unfortunately I have not found the homeopathic melatonin to be effective, while natural melatonin is. If you can't increase your melatonin naturally it is available on prescription from doctors interested in natural hormones. Certain pathologists can measure your level from your saliva.

So, what should I eat?

Well, you now know that coffee, sugar and fatty foods are not good for you, and that fish and vegetables are desirable, so how do you eat as a busy Western woman? It partly depends on your shape. If you are thin or pear shaped with big thighs, you can eat more grains (bread, pasta, rice) than if you are apple shaped and have a big waist.

Apple shaped women can lose some of those waist inches if they get most of their carbohydrates from vegetables. Sugar is *OUT*. Use low GI foods (look up a list on the website: www.glycemicindex. com) or if the food is high GI, don't have too much of it and have it in a meal with protein to slow down its digestion and absorption so it doesn't cause a peak of blood sugar and insulin. *DO* make sure you get enough protein. The recommended daily amount of protein for a sedentary adult is 0.75 gm protein per kilogram of body weight. Children, and adults who are active, need 1 gm protein/kg body weight. For example: one or two eggs, 100 gm tin of fish and a serve of chicken in a day for an average woman. One slice of ham and a salad is not enough protein for lunch. You will be hungry and craving sweet things in an hour or so.

Suggested eating plan for women with endometriosis

I have formulated an eating plan specifically for women with endometriosis using all the dietary factors that research suggests. If you have food cravings on this diet they should settle down after a few days on this eating plan.

Use olive oil for all cooking, rather than sunflower, safflower or canola and definitely do not use mixed vegetable oil. Sprinkle LSA or ground linseed on almost everything. Organic fruit and vegetables with free-range meat and chicken are a good investment.

Breakfasts
- Unsweetened muesli with 2 teaspoons LSA and soy milk or soy yoghurt
- Soy yoghurt and LSA
- Egg and soy linseed toast
- Egg and tomatoes and mushrooms
- 1 or 2 eggs and 2 or 3 of the following: fried pumpkin *or* aubergine slices, *or* mushrooms, steamed broccoli, red capsicum, spinach *or* beetroot tops
- Miso soup with silken tofu (most Japanese women have this every day)
- Tinned kippers and lemon juice on spinach
- Baked beans on soy linseed toast with fresh tomato

Lunches
- Soy linseed roll with salad and tuna, pink salmon, chicken or turkey *or* omit the roll and have at least 100 gm of the meat or fish with salad
- Smoked salmon and avocado in a salad or sandwich
- Takeaway Asian stir-fry with prawns, squid, other seafood
- Homemade soup with chicken and lots of vegetables
- Lebanese falafel and hummus roll with lettuce and tomato and tahini dressing
- Bean salad and lots of other salads. Try sprouts such as lentil, alfalfa or mixed sprouts. Dressings are OK in small amounts

Dinners
- Vegetables and fish — grilled, curried with tomato or coconut milk. Rice is usually eaten with this, but you will be better off with more vegetables instead if you need to lose those waist inches

- Vegetable curry with tinned beans and rice (use plenty of turmeric, onions and garlic in all your cooking)
- Vegetarian dinners with chickpeas, red kidney beans, dhal or lentils
- Veal, chicken, turkey dishes, always with plenty of vegetables
- Lean red meat once a week or less, and not char grilled
- Egg and vegetable frittata — put semi-cooked vegetables in a frying pan with beaten egg. Cook on low heat until the bottom is done then put under the grill for a few minutes. No more than 2 egg yolks per day, but you can use egg whites freely
- Lentil patties and buckwheat and vegetables
- Seafood marinara pasta (use wholemeal spaghetti or 100 per cent durum wheat as they have a lower GI) *and* vegetables

Desserts
- Fresh fruit and yoghurt (soy preferably)
- Diet jelly and pineapple

Snacks
- Fresh pineapple — eat one per week
- Nuts and seeds. The oil they contain is good for us
- Celery and carrot sticks with Lebanese dips — hummus and baba ganoush (made of roasted aubergine). Most other dips are made of cream cheese or pate, which are high in fat
- Apricots, strawberries, plums, half an apple. Most other fruit has a lot of sugar, which will trigger an insulin spike unless it is in small amounts in with a meal
- If you 'need' sweet things, make sure they are at the end of a meal so the other food will slow its absorption and prevent a peak of blood sugar and insulin. Have only a tiny taste, for example 2 squares of chocolate and then put it away!

Won't all this protein cause inflammation?

This diet does not have excess protein. In this eating plan I have combined the anti-inflammatory effects of fish and vegetables with the insulin-reducing effects of lowering carbohydrate and getting sufficient protein. In most people the reduction of sugar and fat will be effective in reducing inflammation and therefore pain. If after a month you still have lots of pain, reduce the arachidonic acid (which prostaglandins are made from) by reducing egg yolks to one per day and making sure the meat has no visible fat, and marinating any red meat in olive oil and red wine for 24 hours in the fridge. Fish and white meats like pork and veal have much less arachidonic acid than red meat.

But does it work? (Sarah's story)

Sarah, age 29, had had endometriosis for seven years. She had a very large tender scar on her abdomen, which was the result of poor wound healing in several operations. I suspected zinc deficiency. She couldn't lie on her tummy or have any pressure on her abdomen. This made it difficult for sex, which was painful inside as well. Her periods were very heavy and painful and so she was on two-month cycles of an oral contraceptive. When off the hormone tablets her breasts were very sore and she had a migraine for the whole five days. (This suggests too much oestrogen.) A previous medication had affected her liver. She had always had chronic flatulence and abdominal discomfort and recently, severe dizzy episodes.

I prescribed progesterone cream, zinc, a liver formula, vitamin C and an organic diet with less bread, and ordered a blood test for iron and gluten intolerance (because of the flatulence and possible zinc deficiency). I also injected the scar with local anaesthetic (lignocaine). This is a treatment from Germany called 'Neural therapy', that helps chronic pain. After a second treatment she had no more pain in the scar.

After two weeks she was feeling better, even though she was in the premenstrual week. She usually had severe PMS and migraine. As the blood test showed she had antibodies to gluten,

I started her on a gluten-free diet (no wheat, rye, oats or barley). A gluten-free diet would not be necessary for most women with endometriosis but in her case it was the reason she was poorly nourished and the aromatase – oestrogen – inflammation cycle was perpetuating itself.

At two months she told me that the gluten-free diet had helped immediately with stomach discomfort and she had more energy. Sexual intercourse was no longer painful. I changed the liver formula to one with soy, red clover and black cohosh, to reduce the effect of oestrogen and help with cramps and PMS.

After five months she said she'd 'never felt healthier'. She had normal bowel actions and no flatulence or cramps. She had only a small headache and a little period cramp on the day before her recent period. She had no dizziness or white spots on her nails since she had been taking zinc, and cold sores were happening less often. These are all linked with low zinc.

After eight months periods were lighter and not so painful. She prefers to remain on the Pill for contraception. She still uses progesterone cream and the female herbs and says she feels 'fantastic'.

Help! It's all too hard!

Well, let's try to summarise what you need to do and form a practical plan. You certainly won't need to do everything I have talked about. I suggest you make a list of the items you think are important for you and then form a plan of action and talk it over with your doctor. My most successful patients keep a folder or book and record the important changes and thoughts about the process. Apparently keeping a diary of your problems and the resulting feelings helps to resolve emotional problems too.

The first steps to get started

- The diet. This is the most important thing, so sit down and make a shopping list of all those foods you are going to need.
- Increase your progesterone. If you're not on the Pill, get some vitex; if you are on the Pill, get a script for natural progesterone cream from a doctor.
- Supplements of zinc 30–50 mg daily (for example zinc chelate 220 mg twice daily).
- Omega 3 fish oil capsules 1000 mg three times daily.
- A multi-vitamin with 25–50 mg of vitamin B6 in the morning. (Actually a multivitamin for men is good if it has the herbs nettle, saw palmetto or epilobium to inhibit aromatase.)
- A women's herbal combination with, for example, soy, red clover and/or black cohosh.

The next steps

- Find a source of organic vegetables, free-range meat and chicken.
- Plan your exercise program – write it down, tell people about it and ask them to encourage you to keep to it. Have your shower after the exercise.
- If you think you have allergies, plan a visit to a natural therapist to get help to work it out.

That will probably be enough for the first month. If you are not improving by then, you will need to adjust the therapy according to the symptoms you still have.

If after a month you still have too much oestrogen, painful periods or new symptoms, you will need to work with your doctor and/or naturopath with the more detailed ideas in this chapter. A trial of chrysin cream, di-indolyl methane, calcium D-glucarate or reduction of progesterone cream may help.

Sadly, there is no one simple pill that will help. Getting the body to resume health is complicated, often needing a significant lifestyle change, but the process is very empowering. You can feel very proud of yourself for managing a complicated condition. Don't forget that in Nature this aromatase – oestrogen – inflammation cycle has its natural controls (otherwise everyone would have endometriosis!) so the answer is to use enough of the natural controls to turn down the speed of the cycle. Thank goodness we have the option of conventional medicine as well.

> I used to think that natural remedies were weak and inefficient compared to prescribed medicines, but now with modern research we know so much about how diet and herbs work that they can be combined scientifically and the results can be stunningly effective.

Chapter 13

....

Conclusion

WHAT WE HAVE WRITTEN in this book is not the end of the story. It is only where we are now. New ways of managing this disease and the other causes of pelvic pain will be found. Some of these new discoveries will prove to be useful. Others will not.

Many of our current treatments will be overtaken by better surgery, better medications, better complementary therapies and better lifestyle advice. We hope to be able to prevent endometriosis altogether one day.

For now, there is the ability to manage pelvic pain better than it has ever been managed before.

Useful websites

The contact details for endometriosis support groups are listed in Chapter 11, on pages 244–45.

In addition, the following websites may be useful for you:

General information on endometriosis
www.ecca.com.au (our clinic website)
www.endocenter.org (USA based website with information and support)
www.endometriosis.org (European website with free email newsletter)
www.endozone.org (the latest news on endometriosis)
www.endo.org.uk (UK National Endometriosis Society)
www.shetrust.org.uk (Endometriosis SHE Trust UK)

Fertility
www.britishfertilitysociety.org.uk
www.fertility.com/australia

Gay health

www.gayhealth.com (a general website with health issues of interest to gay and lesbian couples)

Support for teenagers

www.endocenter.org

www.kidshealth.org (a USA website with health issues for kids and young adults)

Support for men

www.endometriosis.org.uk/partners

www.geocities.com/HotSprings/Spa/8449/eccpartners.html

Counselling

www.bacp.co.uk (British Association for Counselling and Psychotherapy, for information and finding accredited therapists)

Complementary therapies

www.uktherapists.com (UK directory of psychotherapists and comple-amentary therapists)

Other medical conditions

www.ichelp.com (for interstitial cystitis)

www.csp.org.uk (UK Chartered Society of Physiotherapy)

www.physiotherapy.asn.au. The Australian Physiotherapy Association

www.pcos-online.co.uk or www.pcosupport.org (for polycystic ovarian syndrome)

www.menopausematters.co.uk or www.menopause.net.au (for information on menopause and hormone replacement therapy)

www.fpa.org.uk (Family Planning Association)

Glossary

Abdomen
The part of your body that lies between your ribs and the top of your legs.

Adenomyosis
A condition where cells that look like the lining of the uterus are found in the wall of the uterus.

Adhesion
The place where two organs are attached together.

Anti-prostaglandin medications
Medicines that stop the body making chemicals called prostaglandins.

Bilateral salpingo-oophorectomy
An operation to remove the ovaries and fallopian tubes on both sides of the pelvis.

Catheter
A soft rubber tube inserted into the bladder to collect urine.

Cautery
A surgical operation to burn a lesion.

Chocolate cysts
Lumps of endometriosis that are found in one, or both ovaries.

Colostomy
A bowel operation where faeces pass into a bag attached to the abdomen rather than out through the anus.

Cystoscopy
An operation using a thin telescope to view the inside of the bladder.

Danazol
A medication used to treat pain from endometriosis.

Diaphragm
The thin muscle that separates the abdomen from the chest.

Dysmenorrhoea
The medical name for painful periods.

Dyspareunia
The medical name for painful intercourse/sex.

Dysuria
The medical name for pain when passing urine.

Endometriomas
The medical name for chocolate cysts in the ovaries.

Endometrium
The medical name for the lining of the uterus. This is the tissue that bleeds during a period.

Excisional surgery
Surgery to remove endometriosis by 'cutting it out'.

Fibroids
Benign tumours that grow in the muscle wall of the uterus.

Frequency
Passing urine more often than normal.

Gestrinone
A medication used to treat the pain of endometriosis.

GnRH analogue
A medication used to treat the pain of endometriosis.

Hysterectomy
An operation to remove the uterus.

Incision
A skin cut made during an operation.

Laparoscopy
An operation through small holes used to look inside the abdomen.

Laparotomy
An operation through a larger incision used to look inside the abdomen.

Lesion
Any unusual or abnormal area.

Navel
Belly button or umbilicus.

Opioids
Medications to treat pain from any cause.

Ovulation pain
Pain felt when the ovary releases an egg.

Pelvis
The part of your body inside your hip bones.

Peritoneum
The thin slippery skin that covers the pelvic organs.

Speculum
Instrument placed in the vagina to view the cervix and take a smear test.

Symptoms
Things you notice when you are unwell.

Ureter
The tube that carries urine from the kidney to the bladder.

Urethra
The tube that carries urine from the bladder to the outside.

Uterosacral ligaments
These ligaments pass from the uterus back to a part of the spine called the sacrum at the back of the pelvis.

References

The abstracts for these studies can be found at www.ncbi.nlm.nih.gov/
pubmed by searching for the author. For example, to look up reference
number 24, type in Agarwala N, then search.

You will need to go to a medical library if you wish to read the full
article.

1   Donnez, J. & Squifflet, J., *et al. Typical and subtle atypical presentations
    of endometriosis.* OG Clinics of Nth America, 2003 Mar, pp. 83–94.

2   Redwine, D.B. *Ovarian endometriosis: a marker for more extensive
    pelvic and intestinal disease.* Fertil Steril, 72(2): 1999 Aug, pp. 310–5.

3   Husby, G.K., Haugen, R.S. & Moen, M.H., *Diagnostic delay in women
    with pain and endometriosis.* Acta Obstet Gynecol Scand, 82(7), 2003
    Jul, pp. 649–53.

4   Ballweg, M.L. *Endometriosis. The complete reference to taking charge of
    your health.* Contemporary Books, McGraw Hill, USA, 2004, pp. 354–60.

5   Abbott, J., Hawe, J., Hunter, D., Holmes, M., Finn, P. & Garry, R.
    *Laparoscopic excision of endometriosis: a randomized, placebo-
    controlled trial.* Fertil Steril, 82(4), 2004 Oct, pp. 878–84.

6   Demco, L. Mapping of pelvic pain under local anesthesia using
    patient assisted laparoscopy, *Textbook of Laparoscopy*, eds J. Hulka &
    H. Reich. W.B. Saunders Company, Philadelphia, 1998, pp. 391–7.

7   Chapron, C., Pierre, F., Querleu, D. & Dubuisson, J.B. *Complications of
    laparoscopy in gynaecology.* Gynecol Obstet Fertil, 29 (9), 2001 Sep,
    pp. 605–12.

8   Shaw, R.W. (ed.). *Endometriosis. Current understanding and
    management.* Blackwell Science, 1995, pp. 195–201.

9   Moghissi, K.S., Schlaff, W.D., Olive, D.L., Skinner, M.A. & Yin, H.
    *Goserelin acetate (Zoladex) with or without hormone replacement
    therapy for the treatment of endometriosis.* Fertil Steril, 69 (6), 1998
    Jun, pp. 1056–62.

10 Fraser, I.S. & Kovacs, G.T. *The efficacy of non-contraceptive uses for hormonal contraceptives.* MJA, 178 (12), 2003, pp. 621–3.

11 Bulun, S.E., Zeitoun, K., Takayama, K., Noble, L., *et al. Oestrogen production in endometriosis and use of aromatase inhibitors to treat endometriosis.* Endocrine Related Cancer, 6, 1999; pp. 293–301.

12 Vercellini, P., Frontino, G., De Giorgi, O., Aimi, G., Zaina, B., Crosignani, P.G. *Comparison of a levonorgestrel-releasing intrauterine device versus expectant management after conservative surgery for symptomatic endometriosis: a pilot study.* Fertil Steril, 80(2), Aug 2003, pp. 305–9.

13 Fedele, L., Bianchi, S., Zanconato, G., Portuese, A. & Raffaelli, R. *Use of a levonorgestrel-releasing intrauterine device in the treatment of rectovaginal endometriosis.* Fertil Steril, 75(3), 2001 Mar, pp. 485–8.

14 Chatman, D.L. & Ward, A.B. *Endometriosis in adolescents.* J Reprod Med, 27(3), 1982 Mar, pp. 156–60.

15 Abbott, J.A., Hawe, J., Clayton, R.D. & Garry, R. *The effects and effectiveness of laparoscopic excision of endometriosis: a prospective study with 2–5 year follow-up.* Hum Reprod, 18(9), 2003 Sep, pp. 1922–7.

16 Treloar, S. *Genetic influences on endometriosis in an Australian twin sample.* Fertil Steril, 71(4), 1999 Apr, pp. 701–10 and personal communication from S. Treloar.

17 Jansen, R. *Getting Pregnant.* 2nd edn. Allen & Unwin, Sydney, 2003.

18 Van Gorp, T., Amant, F., Neven, P., Vergote, I. & Moerman, P. *Endometriosis and the development of malignant tumours of the pelvis. A review of literature.* Best Pract Res Clin Obstet Gynaecol, 18(2), 2004 Apr, pp. 349–71.

19 Borgfeldt, C. & Andolf, E. *Cancer risk after hospital discharge diagnosis of benign ovarian cysts and endometriosis.* Obstet Gynecol Surv, 59(7), 2004 Jul, pp. 510–11.

20 Davis, S.R., Briganti, E.M., Chen, R.Q., Dalais, F.S., Bailey, M. & Burger, H.G. *The effects of Chinese medicinal herbs on postmenopausal vasomotor symptoms of Australian women. A randomised controlled trial.* Med J Aust, 174(2), 2001 Jan, pp. 68–71.

21 Shepherd, S. & Gibson, P. Unpublished information.

22 Butler, D. & Moseley, G. *Explain Pain.* 2003. Available from www.noigroup.com/ep

23 Belenky, A., Bartal, G., Atar, E., Cohen, M. & Bachar, G.N. *Ovarian varices in healthy female kidney donors: incidence, morbidity, and clinical outcome.* Am J Roentgenol, 179 (3), 2002 Sep, pp. 625–7.

24 Agarwala, N. & Liu, C.Y. *Laparoscopic appendectomy.* J Am Assoc Gynecol Laparosc, 10 (2), 2003 May, pp. 166–8.

25 Hesseling, M.H. & De Wilde, R.L. *Endosalpingiosis in laparoscopy.* J

Am Assoc Gynecol Laparosc, 7(2), 2000 May; pp. 215–9.

26   Thompson, JC & Redwine, DB. Chronic pelvic pain associated with autoimmunity and systemic and peritoneal inflammation and treatment with Immune Modification. J Reprod. Med, 2005 Oct; 50(10): 745–58.

27   King, R. *Good Loving, Great Sex*. Random House, Australia, 1997.

28   Le, M.G., Moulton, L.H., Hill, C. & Kramar, A. *Consumption of dairy produce and alcohol in a case-control study of breast cancer.* J Nat Cancer Inst, 77(3), 1986 Sep, pp. 633–6.

29   Hollingsworth, E. *Better sexual health for women*. Nature & Health, 22(3), 2001, pp. 48–52.

30   Rier, S. & Foster, G.F. *Environmental Dioxins and Endometriosis*. Semin Reprod Med, 2003; pp. 145–54.

31   Schnare, D.W., Denk, G., Shields, M. & Brunton, S. *Evaluation of a Detoxification Regimen for Fat-stored Xenobiotics*. Med Hypoth, 9, 1982, pp. 265–82.

32   Campbell, D.R. & Kurzer, M.S. *Flavonoid inhibition of aromatase enzyme activity in human preadipocytes*. J Steroid Biochem Mol Biol, 46(3), 1993 Sep, pp. 381–8.

33   Schellenberg, R. *Treatment for the premenstrual syndrome with agnus castus fruit extract: prospective, randomised, placebo controlled study.* British Medical Journal, 322, 2001, pp. 134–7.

34   Mathias, J.R., Franklin, R., Quast, D.C., Fraga, N., Loftin, C.A., Yates, L., & Harrison, V. *Relation of endometriosis and neuromuscular disease of the gastrointestinal tract: new insights*. Fertil Steril, 70(1), 1998 Jul, pp. 81–8.

35   Mills, S.Y., Jacoby, R.K., Chacksfield, M. & Willoughby, M. *Effect of a proprietary herbal medicine on the relief of chronic arthritic pain: a double blind study.* British Journal of Rheumatology, 35, 1996, pp. 874–8.

36   Wilson, M.L. & Murphy, P.A. *Herbal and dietary therapies for primary and secondary dysmenorrhoea*. Cochrane Database Syst Rev, (3), 2001, CD002124.

37   Baghurst, K.I. & Dreosti, I.E. *Zinc and magnesium status of Australian adults*. Nutr Res, 11, 1991, pp. 23–32.

Women with scientific or medical training who wish to know more about the causes of pelvic pain are referred to the textbook:

Howard, FM. *Pelvic Pain. Diagnosis and Management*. ISBN 0-7817-1724-8 Lippincott Williams and Wilkins 2000.

Index